Alternatives to Involuntary Death

Timothy Leary

Ronin Publishing, Inc.

Berkeley CA

The cybernetic age offers
a fascinating set of consumer
choices suddenly appear
on the pop-up menu of
The Evolutionary Café.

Alternatives to Involunatry Death

Timothy Leary

ALternatives to InvoLuntary DeaTH

Published by
Ronin Publishing, Inc.
PO Box 22900
Oakland, CA 94609
www.roninpub.com

Production:

Editor:	Beverly A. Potter, Ph.D.
Cover Design:	Beverly A. Potter, Ph.D.
Book Design:	Beverly A. Potter, Ph.D.

Fonts:

FORNicaTOR—CHanK DieSeL
Goudy Old Style—URW Software
Zekton—Ray Larabie

Library of Congress Card Number: 2008942193
Distributed to the book trade by PGW/Perseus

Derived in part from *Chaos & Cyber Culture* with additional content prepared by Beverly Potter

Let's be bold about opening
up a broad spectrum of Club-
Med post-biologic possibilities
of re-creational dying.

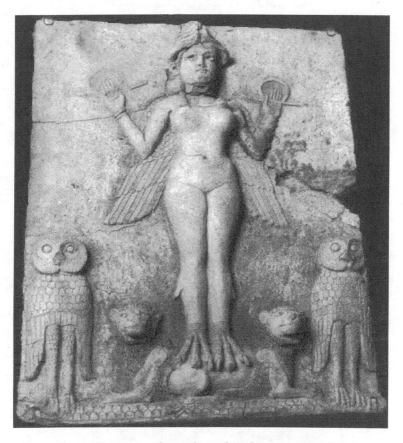

If you expect to be dead when you die,
you will be disappointed.

—PMH ATWATER

You Don't Die

Ronin Books for Independent Minds

by Timothy Leary

High Priest

Chaos & Cyber Culture

The Politics of Ecstasy

Psychedelic Prayers

Change Your Brain

The Politics of Self-Determination

Start Your Own Religion

Your Brain Is God

Turn On Tune In Drop Out

Musings on Human Metamorphoses

Evolutionary Agents

The Politics of PsychoPharmacology

The Fugitive Philosopher

CyberPunks CyberFreedom

Table of Contents

Death is life's greatest event.

—TIMOTHY LEARY

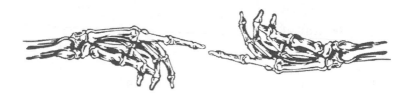

1

THe DYiNG PRocess

m ost human beings face death with an attitude of helplessness, either resigned or fearful. Neither of these submissive, uninformed "angles of approach" to the most crucial event of one's life are ennobling. We've been schooled and counseled—programmed to act out life scripts based on our worst tendencies toward fear and self-doubt.

> I've been looking forward to dying all my life. Dying is the most fascinating experience in life. You've got to approach dying the way you live your life—with curiosity, hope, experimentation, and with the help of your friends.
>
> —TIMOTHY LEARY
> *Design for Dying*

There are many practical options and methods available for navigating the dying process. Passivity, failure to learn about them, might be the ultimate irretrievable blunder. Pascal's famous no-lose wager about the existence of God translates into modern life as a no-risk gamble on the prowess of technology.

Pascal's Wager

Blaise Pascal was a French philosopher, theologian, mathematician and physicist with significant contributions to science. He invented the syringe and helped to create the barometer—an early calculator, as well as contributing to the development of modern probability theory.

Pascal's Wager is a pragmatic rather than an evidential argument for belief in God. The argument presupposes an agnosticism, which is the view that it is impossible to either prove or disprove God's existence.

The theistic tradition holds that our ability to comprehend God is limited because our concepts are derived from our experiences, and our experiences are of flawed and finite existence. Thus we lack the conceptual tools necessary to understand what God is really like.

Pascal argued that because we are unable to determine by reason whether or not God exists, we should base our belief on self-interest. We should play it safe by believing in God and living out a Christian life.

Submission to Authority

For millennia the fear of death has depreciated individual confidence and increased dependence on authority.

True, the loyal members of a familial or racial gene pool can take pride in the successes and survival tenacity of their kinship. For example, around the year 1600, at the height of the obedient, feudal stage Chinese philosopher, Li Zhi, wrote a revealing essay outlining five ways to die.

Five Ways to Die

1. Death for a worthy cause;
2. Death in battle;
3. Death as a martyr;
4. Death as a loyal minister, unjustly attacked;
5. Premature death after finishing some good piece of work.

Thus we see that the aim of the "good life" was one of submission to authority. If your life was dedicated to serving the gene pool, then, logically, your death is the final, crowning sacrifice of your individuality

Instead of treating the last act in your life in terms of fear, weakness, and helplessness, think of it as a triumphant graduation.

—TIMOTHY LEARY
Design for Dying

But for the humanist who believes in the sanctity of the individual, these traditional prospects are less than exalted. Let's be honest here. How can you be proud of your past achievements, walk tall in the present, or zap enthusiastically into the future if, awaiting you implacably around some future corner, is Old Mr. D—the Grim Reaper?

Life is a great sunrise. I do not see why death should not be an even greater one.

—VLADIMIR NOBOKOV

What a PR job the wordmakers did to build this death concept into a primetime horror show! The Grave. Mortification. Extinction. Breakdown. Catastrophe. Doom. Finish. Fatality. Malignancy. Necrology. Obituary. The End.

Note the calculated negativity. To die is to croak, to give up the ghost, to bite the dust, to kick the bucket, to perish. To become inanimate, lifeless, defunct, extinct, moribund, cadaverous, necrotic. A corpse, a stiff, a cadaver, a relic, food for worms, a *corpus delecti*, a carcass. What a miserable ending to the game of life!

> Being born is not a crime, so why must it carry a sentence of death?
>
> —ROBERT ETTINGER

Fear of Death

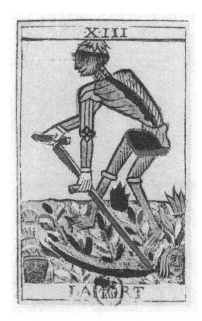

In the past, the reflexive genetic duty of top management— those in social control of the various gene pools—has been to make humans feel weak, helpless, and dependent in the face of death. The good of the race or nation has ensured at the cost of the sacrifice of the individual.

To fear death, gentlemen, is nothing other than to think oneself wise when one is not; for it is to think one knows what one does not know. No man knows whether death may not even turn out to be the greater of blessings for a human being, and yet people fear it as if they knew for certain that it is the greatest of evils.

—SOCRATES

If the flock doesn't fear death, the grip of religious and political management is broken and their power over the gene pool is threatened. When control loosens, dangerous genetic innovations and mutational visions tend to emerge. Obedience and submission were rewarded on a time-payment plan. For our devotion, we are promised immortality in the postmortem hive center variously known as heaven, paradise, or the Kingdom of the Lord. In order to maintain the attitude of dedication, the gene-pool managers had to control the "dying reflexes," orchestrate the trigger stimuli that activate the "death circuits" of the brain. This was accomplished through rituals that imprint dependence and docility when the "dying alarm bells" go off in the brain.

Sperm-Egg Rituals

Perhaps we can better understand this imprinting mechanism by considering another set of "rituals," those by which human hives manage the conception-reproduction reflexes, the fertilization rituals.

Fear of Death Was an Evolutionary Necessity

The mechanisms of control imposed by the operation of social machinery are similar in the two cases. Let us "step outside the system" for a moment, to see vividly what is ordinarily invisible because it is so entrenched in our expectation.

At adolescence each kinship group provides morals, rules, taboos, ethical prescriptions to guide the all-important sperm-egg situation.

Management by the individual of the horny DNA machinery is always a threat to hive inbreeding. Dress, grooming, dating, courtship, contraception, abortion patterns are fanatically conventionalized in tribal and feudal societies. Personal innovation is sternly condemned and ostracized. Industrial democracies vary in the sexual freedom allowed individuals, but in totalitarian states—China and Iran, for example—rigid prudish morality controls the mating reflexes and governs boy-girl relations. Under the Chinese dictator Mao, "romance" was forbidden because it weakened dedication to the state—i.e., the local gene pool. If teenagers pilot and select their own mating, then they will be more likely to fertilize outside the hive, more likely to insist on directing their own lives, and, worst of all, less likely to rear their offspring with blind gene-pool loyalty.

Even more rigid social-imprinting rituals guard the "dying reflexes." Hive control of "death" responses is taken for granted in all pre-cybernetic cultures.

Gene-Pool Protection

In the past, this conservative degradation of individuality was an evolutionary virtue. During epochs of species stability, when the tribal, feudal, and industrial technologies were being mastered and fine-tuned, wisdom was centered in the gene pool, stored in the collective linguistic consciousness, the racial data base of the hive.

Since individual life was short, brutish, aimless, what a singular learned was nearly irrelevant. The world was changing so slowly that knowledge could be embodied only in the breed-culture. Lacking technologies for the personal mastery of transmission and storage of information, the individual was simply too slow and too small to matter. Loyalty to the racial collective was the virtue. Creativity, premature individuation was anti-evolutionary; a weirdo, mutant distraction. Only village idiots would try to commit independent, chaotic, unauthorized thought.

In the feudal and industrial eras, management used the fear of death to motivate and control individuals. Today, politicians use the death-dealing military, the police, and capital punishment to protect the social order.

Among the many things that the pope, the ayatollah, and fundamentalist Protestants agree on is that confident understanding and self-directed mastery of the dying process is the last thing to be allowed to the individual. The very notion of cybernetic post-biologic intelligence or consumer immortality options is taboo, sinful, for formerly valid reasons of gene-pool protection.

Throughout history the priests and mullahs and medical experts have swarmed around the expiring human like black vultures. Death belonged to them.

Rituals help heal the pain of letting go, offering reconciliation and peace, while at the same time connecting us with the divine ... end-of-life rituals can help a person die not only a peaceful death, but also a sacred death.

—MEGORY ANDERSON
Sacred Dying
Creating Rituals for Embracing the End of Life

As we grew up in the 20th Century, we were systematically programmed about how to die. Hospitals are staffed with priests, ministers, and rabbis ready to perform the "last rites." Every army unit has its Catholic chaplain to administer the Sacrament of Extreme Unction—what a phrase, really!—to the expiring soldier. The ayatollah, chief mullah of the Islamic death cult, sends his teenaged soldiers into the Iraq minefields with dog-tags guaranteeing immediate transfer to the Allah's destination resort, Koranic Heaven. A terrible auto crash? Call the medics! Call the priest! Call the reverend!

Organized religion maintains its power and wealth by orchestrating and exaggerating the fear of death.

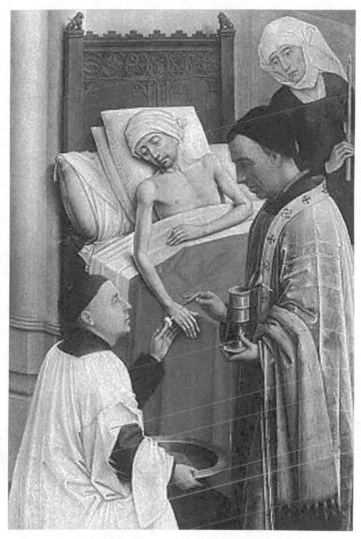

The Seven Sacraments (1445)
by Roger van der Weyden showing
the sacrament of Extreme Unction or
Anointing of the Sick.

Sacrament of Extreme Unction

The Sacrament "Extreme Unction," also called "Last Rites" or "Anointing of the Sick," is the anointing given to those who are gravely ill and those in danger of death from illness or from violence already done to the body. A soldier about to go into battle is not a candidate for the Sacrament, whereas a soldier who has been shot and lies gravely wounded or dying, is entitled to the sacrament.

Religions have cleverly monopolized the rituals of dying to increase control over the superstitious.

The conditions for receiving Unction are that one must have reached the age of reason—usually considered to be around the age of 7, that one be in a state of grace—Penance is part of the Rite, and that one be sorrowful for past sins, trust in God and resign him or herself to God's will, whether to heal the sick person or to will the person's death

The effects of the Sacrament are the strengthening and comfort of the soul of the anointed one, the remission of sins and some of their temporal punishments, and the possible restoration of bodily health.

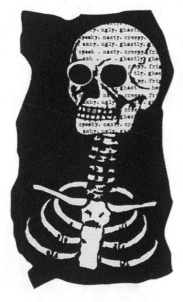

If the flock doesn't fear death, then the grip of religious and political management is broken.

2

FactoRY AssembLY
Line DeatH

In the industrial society, everything becomes part of big business. Dying involves Blue Cross, Medicare, health-care delivery systems, the Health Care Financing Administration (HCFA), terminal patient wards. Undertakers. Cemeteries. The funeral rituals. The monopolies of religion and the assembly lines of top management control the dying and the dead even more efficiently than the living.

For millennia the fear of death has depreciated individual confidence and increased dependence on authority. We recall that knowledge and selective choice about such gene-pool issues as conception, test-tube fertilization, pregnancy, abortion are dangerous enough to the church fathers.

But suicide, right-to-die concepts, euthanasia, life-extension, out-of-body experiences, occult experimentation, astral-travel scenarios, death/rebirth reports, extraterrestrial speculation, cryogenics, sperm banks, egg banks, DNA banks, artificial-intelligence technology—anything that encourages the individual to engage in personal speculation and experimentation with immortality—is anathema to the orthodox seed-shepherds of the feudal and industrial ages.

Why? Because if the flock doesn't fear death, then the grip of religious and political management is broken. The power of the gene pool is threatened. And when control loosens in the gene pool, dangerous genetic innovations and mutational visions tend to emerge.

Age of Individual Responsibility

The cybernetic age we are entering could mark the beginning of a period of enlightened and intelligent individualism, a time unique in history when technology is available to individuals to support a huge diversity of personalized lifestyles and cultures, a world of diverse, interacting, small social groups whose initial-membership number is one.

The exploding technology of light-speed and multimedia communication lays a delicious feast of knowledge and personal choice within our easy grasp. Under such conditions, the operating wisdom and control naturally passes from eons-old power of gene pools, and locates in the rapidly self-modifying brains of individuals capable of dealing with an ever-accelerating rate of change.

Aided by customized, personally programmed, quantum-linguistic appliances, individuals can choose their own social and genetic future, and perhaps choose *not* to "die."

Man is not born free, but everywhere in biological chains. People of the world, unite. You have nothing to lose but your biological chains!

— SIMON YOUNG
Designer Evolution

Wave Theory of Evolution

Current theories of genetics suggest that evolution, like everything else in the universe, comes in waves.

> Humankind is an evolutionary species. Let us then adopt an Evolutionary Ethics: We cannot separate ourselves from the ongoing process of evolution—we *are* evolution.
>
> —SIMON YOUNG
> *Designer Evolution*
> *A Transhumanist Manifesto*

At times of "punctuated evolution," collective metamorphoses, when many things are mutating at the same time, the ten commandments of the "old ones" become ten suggestions. At such times of rapid innovation and collective mutation, conservative hive dogma can be dangerous, suicidal. Individual experimentation and exploration, the thoughtful methodical scientific challenging of taboos, becomes the key to the survival of the gene school.

Punctuated Evolution

Charles Darwin understood that evolution was a slow and gradual process. By gradual, Darwin did not mean "perfectly smooth," but rather, "stepwise," with a species evolving and accumulating small variations over long periods of time until a new species was born. He did not assume that the pace of change was constant, however, and recognized that many species retained the same form for long periods.

If evolution is gradual, there should be a fossilized record of small, incremental changes on the way to a new species. But scientists have been unable to find most of these intermediate forms. Darwin concluded that the fossil record lacked these transitional stages because it was so incomplete.

But in 1972, evolutionary scientists Stephen Jay Gould and Niles Eldridge proposed another explanation, which they called "punctuated equilibrium." That is, species are generally stable, changing little for millions of years. This leisurely pace is "punctuated" by a rapid burst of change that results in a new species and that leaves few fossils behind.

As we enter the cybernetic age, we arrive at a new wisdom that broadens our definition of personal immortality and gene-pool survival: the post-biologic options of the information species. A fascinating set of consumer choices suddenly appear on the pop-up menu of The Evolutionary Café.

Instinctive Will to Evolve

"Evolution" is complexification. "Will" is the ability of the mind to determine behavior—the Will to Evolve is the instinctive drive of a conscious entity to expand its ability in pursuit of every-increasing survivability and well-being.

—SIMON YOUNG
Designer Evolution
A Transhumanist Manifesto

It is beginning to look as though, in the information society, individual human beings can script, produce, direct their own hibernation and re-animation. Dying becomes a "team sport".

Here we face mutation shock in its most panicky form. As we have done in understanding earlier mutations, the first step is to develop a new language. We should not impose the values or vocabulary of the past species on the new cybernetic culture.

Would you let the buzzwords of a preliterate, paleolithic cult control your life? Will you let the superstitions of a tribal-village culture—now represented by the pope and the ayatollah—shuffle you off the scene? Will you let the mechanical, planned-obsolescence tactics of the factory, Blue Cross culture manage your existence?

Darwin: DNA Hitman

Assignment: to destroy Judeo-Christian Theory of creation; liquidate monotheistic architect–God.

Darwin was a chronic user, perhaps an abuser, of a wide variety of opiate drugs prescribed by English physicians in his time. These eased the agonies of his many inexplicable illnesses, which modern biographers tend to regard as psychosomatic. It is usual to explain that Darwin was so often ill because of the psychological stress of his extreme sexual timidity and social shyness. Kenneth Burke, more incisively, has suggested that the great evolutionist, who was the son of a clergymen and the husband of a pious Methodist lady, knew all-too-well the pain, rage and fury his scientific work would cause in Christian nervous systems.

His illnesses, then, were both a self-punishment for his "blasphemy" and a bio-neural dramatization of his self-doubt.

Opium and opium derivatives produce "little death" experiences and suck the user into fibrous, colling vegetative realities. It is part of the junky mystique that each "hit" is an overdose gamble. The Game of Addiction is to come as close as possible to the botanical one-way Exit.

Darwin's insight into the deep-dark regions of vegetative consciousness was due to the fact that he was a confirmed opium addict. Most of the great Victorian poets used opiates and their verse is haunted with the same vegetative death-rebirth-metamorphoses imagery, the same Gothic horror, that Darwin organized so brilliantly and painstakingly into the Theory of Evolution by Natural Selection.

Darwin was an obsessively dedicated scientist, a hard worker of heroic endurance. It is recorded that

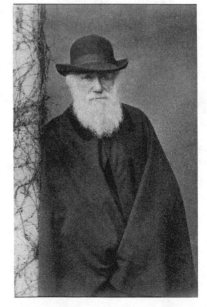

when dissatisfied with some details in his interpretation of barnacle evolution, he laid aside all other work and remorselessly concentrated on barnacles for nearly seven years. His youngest son, assuming this was the normal male role, once asked a neighbor's child, "What sort of barnacles does you father work on?"

At the point of near-death, or in the opiate

quasi-death, vast evolutionary perspec-
tives often appear. We define this as the
seventh circuit of the nervous system.

Dying is a team sport.

Darwin has been proven right on many
points where his actual scientific evidence was wrong
or inadequate. We suggest that his seventh circuit
neurogenetic visions guided him almost as well as his
careful scientific research. Most biographers stress his
love for and empathy with all forms of life. His book
on worms, behind its objective style, has all the ten-
derness of a popular dog story for children.

Darwin: Male Chauvinist Prig

The obvious and deliberate flaw of the Darwinian
theory is caused by its obvious sexual bias. Darwinians
are male chauvinists prigs. We can understand and
sympathize with their problem. It was their exciting
duty to introduce scientific evidence, which changed
orthodox cosmology of the times. For two thousand
years the Judeo-Christian hive-collective had brutality
imposed a barbarous theory of creation. The cosmology held by a hive, i.e., its theory of creation is the basic structure which unifies and organizes the Egg Collective. To link-up and manage the large multi-tribe
collective necessary to produce an industrial society it
was necessary to impose monotheism. Thus a simple-
minded, crude shepherd Jewish tribe divinity was ele-
vated to cosmic importance. The peevish, suspicious,
macho paranoid Jehovah exhibited all the character-
istics of a male-monotheist-monomaniac god: hatred
of women, frantic controlitis, jealous territorial posses-
siveness, intolerance of diversity.

The Judeo-Christian model was organized to op-pose the Egg-Wisdom of the tribal matriarchies. A Gaia Mother Goddess lovers all Her creatures equally and playfully produces new off-spring designed to stimulate and change the older, Egg-Wisdom is the Pantheistic wisdom of change and diversity.

The Darwinians were obsessed with and paralyzed by the Male-Mono-manic divinity. Like Freud, Dar-win was Robot-wired to replace the Father with the new Socialist-Brother Cosmology-Science. But Dar-win and Freud were too timid to burst out of the hive and allow an untidy Egg-Pluralism. So they replaced the Bible with another Male Model—grim chance, natural selection, struggle for existence, survival of the fittest. The key error here was the elimination of creative-intelligence, egg-wisdom, genetic design. To avoid a creator the Darwinians invented the bleak philosophy of meaninglessness. We were created by blind chance! We evolve via copying errors and we are going no where and we are alone and isolated be-cause chance could not have replicated us elsewhere! Hatch as catch can!

It was this benign, compassionate pre-planned concept of evolution, which the Darwinian scientists of the 19th-20th centuries could not handle.

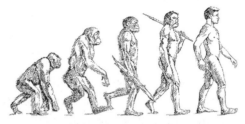

To avoid a creator the Darwinians invented the bleak philosophy of meaninglessness.

3

Re-Creational Dying

T here are commonsense, easy-to-understand options for dealing with death planfully, playfully, compassionately, and elegantly with the inevitable final scene. Thinking for ourselves, we can direct and control our final moments of awareness, reaching that level of meaning and understanding variously referred to as illumination, liberation, and enlightenment. If you're prepared, if you're practiced and practiced then your mind will be free from constricting games that comprise your personality and the hallucinations and fear that often accompany the dying process.

You must understand and accept the dying process as one of total liberation. Conversely failure to accept the responsibility for designing your dying might be the ultimate irretrievable, final victimization. No matter how you've lived your life, in death you are given a chance that mustn't be denied.

Let us explore the option of re-creational dying. For starters, let's demystify dying and develop alternative metaphors for consciousness leaving the body. Let us speculate good-naturedly about post-biologic options. Let's be bold about opening up a broad spectrum of Club-Med post-biologic possibilities. Let us explore the option of re-creational dying.

Our society has tried to make death invisible, thinking that if we ignore it long enough it will go away.

—MEGORY ANDERSON
Sacred Dying

Metabolic Coma

For starters, let's replace the word death with the more neutral, precise, scientific term: *metabolic coma.* And then let's go on to suggest that this temporary state of coma might be replaced by auto-metamorphosis, a self-controlled change in bodily form where the individual chooses to change his or her vehicle of existence without loss of consciousness.

Very few of the superstitions that biologists and medical doctors believe about aging, immortality, and death are true.

—MICHAEL R. ROSE
Biological Immortality
The Scientific Conquest of Death

Then, let's distinguish between involuntary and voluntary metabolic coma. Reversible and irreversible dying. Let's explore those fascinating borderlands—the periods between body dying and neurological dying and DNA dying in terms of the knowledge-information processing involved.

Descartes' "*cognito ergo sum*"—I think therefore I am—signifies the brain's recognition of its own existence distinct from the body. The evolution of the human mind has allowed us to wake up to the horror of our slavery to a genetic program for self-destruction.

—SIMON YOUNG
Designer Evolution
A Transhumanist Manifesto

Let's collect some data about that even more intriguing zone now beginning to be researched in the cross-disciplinary field of scientific study known as artificial life. What knowledge-information-processing capacities can be preserved after both body death and brain cessation? What natural and artificial systems, from the growth of mineral structures to the self-reproduction of formal mathematical automata, are promising alternative candidates to biology for the support of life?

We recognize that the dying process, which for millennia has been blanked by taboo and primitive superstition, has suddenly become accessible to human intelligence.

Let us have no more pious, wimpy talk about death. The time has come to talk cheerfully and joke sassily about personal responsibility for managing the dying process.

And then let us perform the ultimate act of human intelligence. Let's venture with calm, open-minded tolerance and scientific rigor into that perennially mysterious unknown land—a *terra incognita*—and ask the final question: What knowledge-information-processing possibilities can remain after the cessation of all biological life: somatic, neurological, and genetic?

The process of dying is a difficult one, with many fears and anxieties, but it is also a very mysterious and wondrous process. It involves both the body and the soul in the greatest transition we are ever called to make.

—MEGORY ANDERSON
Sacred Dying

How can human consciousness be supported in digital, light-wave, zero-one wafers outside the moist envelope of graceful, attractive, pleasure-filled meat we now inhabit? How can the organic, carbon-constructed caterpillar become the silicon butterfly?

The boundaries between life and death are at best shadowy and vague. Who shall say where one ends and where the other begins?

—EDGAR ALLEN POE

There is no precise moment of death. Instead forensic scientists use clues for estimating the time of death. The first clue, of course, is lack of a pulse.

Signs of Death

1. Heart stops beating and/or lungs stop breathing.

2. Body cells no longer receive supplies of blood and oxygen. Brain cells can die if deprived of oxygen for more than three minutes. Blood drains from capillaries in the upper surfaces and collects in the blood vessels in the lower surfaces. Upper surfaces of the body become pale and the lower surfaces become dark.

3. Cells eventually die and the body loses its capacity to fight off bacteria. Muscle cells live on for several hours. Bone and skin cells can stay alive for several days.

4. Cells cease aerobic respiration and are unable to generate the energy molecules needed to maintain normal muscle biochemistry. Calcium ions leak into muscle cells preventing muscle relaxation. *Rigor mortis*, which is a stiffening of the muscles, sets in after three hours and lasts until 36 hours after death.

   After a body has died, the chemical reaction producing these energy molecules is unable to proceed because of a lack of oxygen. The cells no longer have the energy to pump calcium out of the cell and so the calcium concentration rises, forcing the muscles to remain in a contracted state. This state of muscle stiffening is known as *rigor mortis* and it remains until the muscle proteins start to decompose.

5. The cells' own enzymes and bacterial activity cause the body to decompose and the muscles lose their stiffness.

6. It takes around 12 hours for a human body to be cool to the touch and 24 hours to cool to the core.

Post-Biological Awareness

We recognize that the dying process, which for millennia has been blanketed by taboo and primitive superstition, has suddenly become accessible to human intelligence.

Rage, Rage Against Dying

Do not do gentle into that good night,

Old age should burn and rave at close of day;

Rage, rage, against the dying of the
light.

—DYLAN THOMAS

Here we experience the sudden insights that we need not "go quietly" and passively into the dark night or the neon-lit, enhanced Disney-Heaven of the Jesus Corporation. We realize that the concept of involuntary, irreversible metabolic coma known as "death" is a lethal, feudal superstition, a cruel marketing tactic of industrial society. We understand that one can discover dozens of active, creative alternatives to going belly-up clutching the company logo of the Christian Cross, Blue Cross, or Crescent Cross, or the eligibility cards of the Veterans Administration.

Soliloquy On Death

To be, or not to be,—that is the question
   Whether 't is nobler in the mind to suffer
The slings and arrows of outrageous for-
   tune,
Or to take arms against a sea of troubles,
And, by opposing, end them?—To die, to
   sleep;—
No more; and, by a sleep, to say we end
The heart-ache, and the thousand natural
   shocks
That flesh is heir to,—'t is a consummation
Devoutly to be wished. To die,—to sleep;—
To sleep! perchance to dream:—ay, there's
   the rub;
For in that sleep of death what dreams
   may come,
When we have shuffled off this mortal
   coil,
Must give us pause: there 's the respect
That makes calamity of so long life;
For who would bear the whips and scorns
   of time,
The oppressor's wrong, the proud man's
   contumely,
The pains of despised love, the law's delay,
The insolence of office, and the spurns
That patient merit of the unworthy takes,
When he himself might his quietus make
With a bare bodkin? who would fardels
   bear,

To grunt and sweat under a weary life,
But that the dread of something after
    death,—
The undiscovered country, from whose
    bourn
No traveller returns,—puzzles the will,
And makes us rather bear those ills we
    have,
Than fly to others that we know not of?
Thus conscience does make cowards of
    us all;
And thus the native hue of resolution
Is sicklied o'er with the pale cast of
    thought;
And enterprises of great pith and mo-
    ment,
With this regard, their currents turn
    awry,
And lose the name of action.

—SHAKESPEARE
Hamlet

Recognition is always the beginning of the possibility for change. Once we comprehend that "death"
can be defined as a problem of knowledge-information
memory processing, solutions to this age-long "problem" can emerge.

We realize that the intelligent thing to do is to try
to keep one's knowledge-processing capacities around
as long as possible. In bodily form. In neural form.
In DNA form. In the silicon circuitry and magnetic
storage media of today's computers. In molecular form,

through the atom-stacking of nanotechnology in to-morrow's computers. In cryogenic form. In the form of stored data, legend, myth. In the form of offspring who are cybernetically trained to use post-biologic intelli-gence. In the form of post-biological gene pools, info-pools, advanced viral forms resident in world computer networks and cyberspace matrices of the sort described in the "sprawl novels" of William Gibson.

It is a loathsome and cruel trick that nature takes such an exquisitely won-drous creation as the human brain and imprisons it inside the weak, inefficient, fragile, and short-lived structure that is the human body. Our bodies may be beautiful, but they are unacceptably ephemeral.

—MIKE TREDER
Emancipation From Death
The Scientific Conquest of Death

The second step in attaining post-biologic, re-cre-ational awareness is to shill from the passive to the active mode. Industrial-age humans were trained to await docilely the onset of termination, and then to turn over their body for disposal to the priests and the factory—hospital—technicians.

Our species is now developing the cybernetic information skills and the activists' confidence to plan ahead, to make one's will and testament prevail. The smart thing to do is to see dying as a change in the implementation of information processing: to orches-trate it, manage it, anticipate and exercise the many available options.

Star Trek Philosophy is the essence of
humanism: The belief in the ongoing
progress of the species through reason,
science, and technology. Without the in-
stinct to progress, humankind is doomed
to remain forever at the mercy of the
disease, decay, and the limitations of the
human body and mind.

—SIMON YOUNG
Designer Evolution
A Transhumanist Manifesto

Recognition is always
the beginning of the
possibility for change.

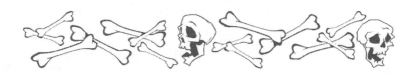

4

DEMYSTIFY DYING

T he time has come to talk cheerfully and joke sassily about personal responsibility for managing the dying process. For starters, let's demystify dying and develop alternative metaphors for consciousness leaving the body. Let us speculate good-naturedly about post-biologic options. Let's be bold about opening up a broad spectrum of Club-Med post-biologic possibilities. Let us explore the option of re-creational dying.

> The house party is a wonderful way to deal with your divinity as you approach death. I can't recommend it enough ....
> You can write the programs for how you will de-animate.
> —TIMOTHY LEARY
> *Design for Dying*

The circuits of the brain that mediate the "dying" process are routinely experienced during "near-death" crises. For centuries people have reported: "My entire life flashed before my eyes as I sank into the water."

This "near-death, out-of-body" experience can be turned on via certain aesthetic drugs—Ketamine, for example. Or by learning enough about the effects of out-of-body drugs so that one can use hypnotic techniques to activate the desired circuits without using external chemical stimuli.

Near-Death Experiences

Polls show that more than thirteen million Americans have had a near-death experience (NDE) where they clinically died, or came close to death, and then were revived.

Many people report that during this limbo period they encounters with spirit guides, seeing dead relatives or friends, feelings of total serenity, security, or warmth life review, detachment from the body, the presence of light, which seems like a deity or spiritual presence, or a moment of decision where they are able to decide or are told to turn back.

Near-death experiences suggest that consciousness exists beyond death. Near-death stories passing through a dark tunnel, then refocusing and becoming aware of a detached spiritual body watching the physical body with revival efforts underway. Subsequently a world filled with light and freedom emerges in which the individual meets a "being of light" who portrays perfect understanding and love, leaving them with a deep sense of peace and well-being.

Ancient Egyptians believed that each individual had two souls, a *ba* and a *ka*, which separated at death unless steps were taken to prevent this division. Egyptian descriptions of the *ba* and *ka* are strikingly similar to modern scientists' descriptions of the conscious and unconscious halves of the human psyche.

Many other cultures all over the globe believe in two souls, one like the conscious, the other like the unconscious, which separated at death. Many cultures hold that one soul would go on to reincarnate, while the other would become trapped in a dreamlike netherworld. Some believe that this division could be prevented or reversed, while others see the division as being inevitable. The two stages of near-death experiences—a detached, objective, and dispassionate black void followed by a subjective, relationship-oriented, and emotionally intense realm of light—reflect the distinctions between the conscious mind and the unconscious mind. The darkness stage seems to be experienced exclusively through the conscious half of the psyche, while the light stage seems to be experienced exclusively through the unconscious, as if the two were operating independently during these episodes.

A similarly polarized dichotomy can be found in the accounts of reincarnation, of the Realm of Bewildered Souls, of the void between lives, of the behavior of ghosts and apparitions, and in statements about the afterlife by parapsychologists. The Binary Soul Doctrine hypothesis—that the two halves of the psyche separate after death—offers a consistent explanation for these afterlife phenomena.

We see immediately that the rituals intuitively developed by religious groups are designed to induce hypnotic-trance states related to "dying." The child growing up in a Catholic culture is deeply imprinted—programmed—by funeral rites. The arrival of the solemn priest to administer extreme unction becomes access codes for the pre-mortem state. Other cultures have different rituals for activating and then controlling—programming—the death circuits of the brain. Until recently, very few have permitted personal control or customized consumer choice.

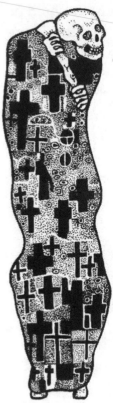

Almost every animal species manifests "dying reflexes." Some animals leave the herd to die alone. Others stand with legs apart, stolidly postponing the last moment. Some species eject the dying creature from the social group.

Death Rattle

There are many symptoms that indicate that we are approaching our death. One of the most well-known is the *death rattle*. The death rattle is a sound that is produced when air moves through mucus that has accumulated in the throat of a dying person after loss of the cough reflex and loss of the ability to swallow. This is a very common symptom, though it does not always occur prior to death. The death rattle does not cause any discomfort to the patient, however, family members frequently find the sound disturbing.

The death rattle is an indication that death is very near. This type of breathing may go on for hours, but usually the patient will die within 24 hours of onset.

Navigational Control of Dying

To gain navigational control of one's dying processes, three steps suggest yourself: First, activate the death reflexes imprinted by your culture, experience them. Imagine dressing up like a priest, rabbi, or minister and mimic their solemn, hypnotic rituals. Visualize. Recite the prayers for the dying. Do these things in the virtual reality of your mind. Officiate at your own platonic funeral. Second, trace your origins. And, third, reprogram, install your own pre-mortem plan for immortality.The aim is to develop a scientific model of the chain of cybernetic—knowledge-information—processes that occurs as one approaches this metamorphic stage and to intentionally develop options for taking active responsibility for these events.

All Things Pass

All things pass

A sunrise does not last all morning

All things pass

A cloudburst does not last all day

All things pass

Nor a sunset all night.

But Earth . . . sky . . . thunder . . .

wind . . . fire . . . lake . . .

Mountain . . . water . . .

These always change.

And if these do not last

Do man's visions last?

Do man's illusions?

During the season

Take things as they come.

All things pass.

From Psychedelic Prayers
& Other Meditations

5

Achieving Immortality

Here we are, the first species that's ever effectively taken over its own evolution .... It's like human evolution is now designer evolution.

—WILLIAM GIBSON

Since the dawn of human history, philosophers and theologians have speculated about immortality. Uneasy, aging kings have commanded methods for extending the life span.

A most dramatic example of this age-long impulse is ancient Egypt, which produced mummification, the pyramids, and manuals like the *Book of the Dying*.

The Tibetan Book of the Dying presents a masterful Buddhist model of post-mortem stages and techniques for guiding the student to a state of immortality,

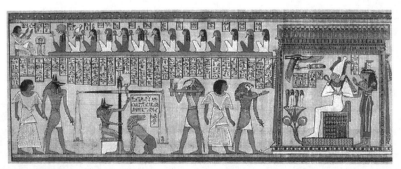

which is neurologically "real" and suggests scientific techniques for reversing the dying process.

The new field of molecular engineering is pro-ducing techniques within the framework of current consensus Western science to implement auto-meta-morphosis. The aim of the game is to defeat death—to give the individual mastery of this, the final stupidity.

We do not endorse any particular technique of achieving immortality. Our aim is to review all op-tions and encourage creative thinking about new possibilities.

Brain Preservation

There are three scientific methods for pre-serving the hardware of the brain after physical death.

1. Cloning a new brain and body from cells.
2. Cryonic suspension of the body and/or brain.
3. Biological brain banking—awaiting donor transplant to a new body.

Preserving the brain does not assure that the soft-ware directories, the memory files and the personal operating systems, will be preserved. Therefore, the owner of the brain must make arrangements to "save" and "back up" the memory software that comprises the individual's personality and consciousness of self.

The brain is an organic computer. The
human mind is a brain that recognizes
its own existence.

—SIMON YOUNG
Designer Evolution
A Transhumanist Manifesto

Storing personal memories and genetic algorithms
in the brain to be backed up and stored for uploading
into the new or re-animated brain.

Owners who wish to preserve and re-animate their
neuro-memories—souls—must diligently collect and
protect material mementos that will help reconstruc-
tion the unique personality and personal environment
of their lives—within reason. The tombs of pharaohs
are models of personal-reality storage, but impracti-
cal for our times. Material items, mementos, souve-
nirs, clothes,
books, and
pictures are
obviously
vulnerable to
loss. The key
to software
backup is
digitization.

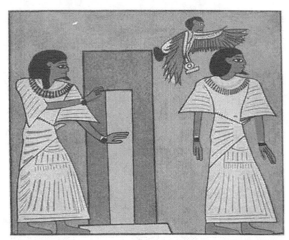

THE SOUL COMES FORTH FROM THE TOMB

6

Re-CRealional Alternatives to Involuntary Irreversible Metabolic Coma

There are a variety of techniques useful in experiencing "experimental dying," reversible-voluntary exploration of the territory between body coma and brain death, sometimes called out-of-body experiences; or near-dying experiences. Others have termed these experiences astral travel or reincarnation memories

> Leary took every opportunity to let people know that we have choices regarding how to die and, someday soon, we may have choices about *whether* to die.

> —R.U. SIRIUS
> *Design for Dying*

Meditation and Hypnosis

The classic yogic routes to exploration of non-ordinary states of consciousness, well-known to be labor- and time-intensive. Out of body experiences seem to be

reserved for dying people or monks with ten plus years
of intense meditation practice have. The aim is to at-
tain an out-of-body experience, which involves a sensation of floating outside of one's body and perceiving
one's physical body from a place outside one's body.

Now there is a fast-track to getting out of our bodies. In his book, *Adventures Beyond the Body: Proving
Your Immortality Through Out-Of-Body Travel,* William Buhlman outlines basic steps for stimulating
an out-of-body experience. First is to use meditative
techniques to get into a light trance state, which is expanded into a vibrational state, where you feel vibrations pulsating through your body. The final step is
separating your astral body from the physical body.

Enthusiasts of Bhulman's method report that
it generally takes about two weeks of following his
techniques to wake up in the dream state, climb out of
your body and walk around your apartment.

Psychedelic Experiences

Re-creational—psychedelic—drugs can be used to
access information and operational programs stored in
the brain of the individual. In normal states of consciousness, these states are not available for voluntary access.

Aldous Huxley was ardently interested in both the
dying experience and its parallels in the religious and
mystical experiences induced by psychedelic drugs.
Huxley used a hypnotic technique to bring his dying
wife, Maria, into touch with the memory of ecstatic
experiences that had occurred spontaneously on several occasions during her life, by guiding her toward

these mystical states of consciousness as death was approaching.

In a letter to Humphry Osmond, a psychiatrist and pioneer in psychedelic research who introduced him to LSD and mescaline, Huxley wrote: "My own experience with Maria convinced me that the living can do a great deal to make the passage easier for the dying, to raise the most purely physiological act of human existence to the level of consciousness and perhaps even of spirituality."

In Huxley's future vision, *Brave New World*, "soma" and the "moksha medicine" in *Island* are psychedelic substances similar to LSD, mescaline, and psilocybin that facilitate insights that free us from the fear of death and enable us to live more fully.

Huxley's second wife, Laura, relayed that he believed that "the last rites should make one more conscious rather than less conscious, more human rather than less human." Several hours before Huxley's death in 1963 he asked Laura to give him 100 micrograms of LSD to facilitate his own dying, which she described in *This Timeless Moment*.

All human beings, all persons who reach adulthood in the world today are programmed biocomputers. None of us can escape our own nature as programmable entities. Literally, each of us may be our programs, nothing more, nothing less.

—JOHN C. LILLY, M.D.
Programming the Human BioComputer

What John Lilly calls metaprogramming agents in his ground-breaking book, *Programming and Metaprogramming in The Human Biocomputer*—these electro-chemical imprints—can be re-programmed, or re-imprinted. Lilly described this ability to re-program

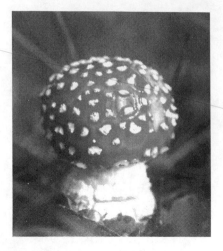

our programs, meta-programs, then goes into considerable scientific and rigorous detail describing all the ways we can metaprogram our own brains, changing our programming as we see fit.

In the province of the mind, what the mind believes to be true, either is true or becomes true within certain limits to be found experientially and experimentally. These limits are further beliefs to be transcended. In the mind there are no limits.

—JOHN C. LILLY. M.D.
The Scientist

Even though in the mind there are no limits, the body on the planet-side trip has definite limits locked in by biology. So as long as we return to and operate within it, we are subject to its limits. However each day we are becoming more aware of how these genetic limits work, and soon will figure out how to overcome those limits, first with genetic engineering, then nanoengineering.

Ketamine

Carefully designed for experimental out-of-body experiences. John Lilly wrote extensively about his experiences with small dosages of anesthetics such as Ketamine. It is possible that the out-of-body subjective effects of such substances are interpretations of proprioceptive disruption.

Ketamine hydrochloride is a fast-acting, hallucinogenic, "dissociative" general anesthetic used in surgical procedures on both animals and humans. Ketamine is a powerful entheogen with the capacity to generate inner experiences of God, gods, and divinity. Many people consider ketamine, or K, to a shamanic experience hat gives deeper understanding of our role in the universe.

The ketamine experience is often death-like with an external sensory shutdown and a move toward an inner universe to reach a transcendental experience of "oneness". Many using K say that during their experience they felt that they understood the Christian notion of the separation of the soul and the body and that they came to believe some part of them will continue to exist after death. Many reported direct contact with God in the form of an ocean of brilliant white light filled with love, bliss and energy.

K tends to stimulate near-death experiences with a feeling of leaving the body to have a sense of timelessness and feeling of calm and peace.

Ketamine is a deceptively dangerous drug because of the high probability of addiction and has been called the "Frankenstein molecule." K addicts have been known to die during the experience. DM Turner, an experienced psychonaut who claimed to have had more than 100 K trips, is believed to have drowned in a bath tub while using ketamine on New Year's Eve.

Laughing Gas or nitrous oxide (N^2O) is a similar analgesic used in dentistry for pain control that yields similar perceptual experiences but for a much shorter time per does—generally 30 second or so. Thus, it is vastly less dangerous so long as the tripper has sufficient access to oxygen.

Sensory deprivation

Dr. John Lilly's research showed that metaprogramming of our beliefs and programs can be accomplished in a state of sensory isolation. Lilly created an "isolation tank," which is a lightless, soundproof tank in which a person floats in salty water at skin temperature.

To study your mind, it must be isolated from sensory stimulation and from of reaction in the here-and-now external reality. To achieve this Lilly devised the "void method" using the sensory isolation tank in which he studied the workings of his mind. Lilly showed that an isolated mind can study its own processes, free of feedback with the external world.

Relaxation

Physical restoration can be accelerated through the use of flotations therapy. When floating the body reaches states of total relaxation where tension is released and the energy is allowed to flow into the needed areas. When the burden of processing is reduced, the body has access to immense resources to heal itself. This healing energy is intelligent, needs no direction, and prioritizes according to ones personal needs.

Lilly discovered that when he cut off sensory input he become aware that his Self was programmed by program systems he had not been aware of in daily external reality. He said, "I discovered that I am something and someone far greater than my simulation of my Self."

Your Metabelief Operator is clearest in a void or isolation environment.

—JOHN C. LILLY, M.D.
The Quiet Center

A phenomenon called deautomatization occurs while floating. The body is automated, which enables us to accomplish tasks without consciously processing each action every time. Automatization can produce unwanted effects, which include habits, compulsion, and tension. These habit patterns can lead to medical problems such as digestive ailments and cancer.

When floating, the mind/body system realizes that the normal stimulus has decreased dramatically, which causes the system to turn up the "volume" for the sensing of available stimulus. In the sensory deprivation environment the mind/body system proceeds to reset its muscle memory, which is one of the reasons that people emerge from the flotations tanks totally relaxed and experience more vivid colors, more flavor, and a general state of heightened awareness.

If you are around in 2010 you will have an excellent chance to live to the year 2030. If you are around in 2030—regardless of your age—you will be able to live indefinitely into the future.

—FM-2030
Are You a Transhuman?

If the human race took death seriously, there would be no more of it.

—CELIA GREEN

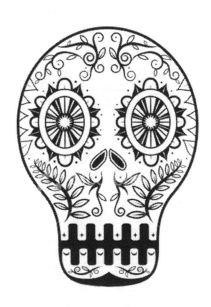

7

Life Extension Diet

The classic approach to immortality has been to inhibit the process of aging comprise. In the present state of science, these serve to buy time. Take brain health seriously. Protect your head. The classic research on diet and longevity was done by Roe L. Walford, M.D. as reported in his book, *The 120-Year Diet: Maximum Life Span*.

Roy Walford

Roy Walford, M.D., a professor in the Department of Pathology, School of Medicine, University of California at Los Angeles. In addition to his teaching, laboratory work, and publishing, Walford did field work in the Amazon jungle, studying the immunology of the Tukuna Indians. He was the physician and medical researcher for the Biosphere 2 in Oracle, Arizona—a major experiment in the early 1990s that involved humans living in a closed-cycle ecological system for several years. It serves as a model for space colonization and sustainable Earth systems.

Early in his career, Walford became interested in autoimmune reaction—an immune reaction to one's self—as a significant cause of aging. During this early stage, Walford pursued research in gerontology where he attempted to analyze which aspects of the immune system decline with time and are directly associated with the aging process. Walford pursued the idea of maximum life span as a parameter to evaluate biological phenomena. Around 1974, he also developed an interest in how the immune system functions within a situation of life-span extension.

Walford's interest grew in the idea of using the life-extension model for determining which biological systems are critical to aging. He asserted that the maximum genetic life span must have been extended by retarding the aging process. Therefore by monitoring biological systems during a caloric-restriction experiment, it can be determined which systems are critical to aging. Those systems that continue to decline along their normal trajectory are not critical. Those systems that do not decline along their normal trajectory are probably the ones responsible for the life extension.

Take Supplements

Always take a good multivitamin supplement when on a calorie restriction diet. Theoretically it is possible to obtain all the vitamins and micronutrients you need from your food. But in practice, most of us don't get all of the vitamins and nutrients that we need—especially when on a caloric restrictive diet.

Eat Brain Foods

Food that is good for the heart is also good for the brain. Eat food high in antioxidants such as food and vegetables, which reduce inflammation by 50%. Inflammation is associated with disease.

Take Vitamin E and C, which are antioxidants that, according to Dr. Daniel Amen, brain health specialist, reduces inflammation by 68%. Eat the brain food, fish, which is high in DNA, and olive oil which is high in Vit E.

Curcumin

Gerontologist Steve Harris, M.D. notes that in India the dementia caused by Alzheimer's and senility is about half to a quarter of that of the so-called developed world. Many researchers believe that this is due to the large amounts of curcumin is the main component of turmic and used in curries, a staple of Indian diets. Curcumin appears to be an amazing natural neuroprotectant, at least as good for your brain as DHA/fish oils, and perhaps even better.

UCLA Alzheimer's researcher Greg Cole, Ph.D. Dr. Cole has systematically explored potential Alzheimer's prevention drugs including supplements like DHA, NSAIDs, vitamin E, and many others, as well as the etiology and pathophysiology of neurodegeneration.

Animal trials with curcumin revealed that it has a powerful protective effect against the emergence of mental problems. Curcumin is the only known therapy other than caloric restriction (discussed next) that reliably extends lifespan (about 10-12%) in laboratory mice. Researchers believe that curcumin's life extension effect is due to improved total body immunity—mediated, as with most things, through the brain—in old age.

According to Sally Frautschy, Ph.D. a 900mg curcumin capsule is equal to about five turmeric curry dinners. Curcumin should be taken with food to avoid an upset stomach. Taking it with fatty food, or with a fish oil supplement maximizes absorption.

Eat Less; Live Longer

Gluttony and greed are the killer addictions. Skinny folks live much longer. Eating less as a method of extending life span is called variously "caloric restriction," "dietary restriction," or more currently, "energy restriction." Energy restriction is technically accurate because what is being restricted is the energy content of food, rather than specific nutrients. Even though the amount of energy consumed in food is restricted, there is no lack of energy or lethargy state.

Caloric restriction slows aging and extends the maximum life span. This has been proven by research from Walford and other scientists. In controlled research, caloric restriction has demonstrated maximum increase in the life span of animals. In some cases the increase has been dramatic—almost doubling. Scientists agree: Caloric restriction works in mice, rates, bats. Hamsters, dogs and cats. It works in insects, fish and even microorganisms. After a century of research and several hundred controlled studies, caloric restriction has been shown to be effective in increasing maximum life span in virtually every case where it has been used.

From his research in caloric restriction and immunology, in 1986 Walford wrote *The 120-Year Diet: How to Double Your Vital Years*, where he reviews the scientific work. He makes the case that it will work in humans and prescribes a restricted diet that he uses himself. A leading nutritionist wrote a critical review of the book, stating that the idea of 120 years of life was outrageous. Walford's reputation as a scientist was so conservative that the reviewer speculated the book's title was forced on him by the publisher for advertising purposes. But Walford immediately published a rebuttal in an editorial letter. He rebuked the critic politely but curtly, saying that the reviewer obviously had not read the book. If he had he would have known that 120 years was precisely and literally what Walford meant.

The Hunza

The people of the Hunza do not consciously follow any special diet. . .they eat two meals a day, drink glacier water, and mix work with exercise and pleasure. They do not contaminate their soil. Occasionally, they run out of food at the end of the winter season. Until the new crop is available they have practically nothing to eat, and water has to suffice. Apparently it nourishes them well and they easily survive the period of near starvation. We would call it fasting.

—RENÉE TAYLOR
The Hunza-Yoga Way to Health and Longer Life

A caloric restriction diet aims to reduce your intake of calories to a level 20-40% lower than is typical, while still obtaining all the necessary nutrients and vitamins.

Controlled studies using humans as subjects have yet to be conducted. The people of the Hunza are an isolated group of people who practice caloric restriction by necessity and allegedly live remarkably long, healthy lives. Scientific verification is difficult to obtain from societies that do not use record-keeping practices such as birth certificates, but the average life span of these people is reputedly over a hundred years. By eating only two frugal meals a day and fasting for several weeks at the end of winter, these people are modern-day exemplars of caloric restriction.

Caloric Reduction Case History

Luigi Cornaro was a Venetian nobleman who lived from 1464 to 1565—101 years. At forty Cornaro was destroying his health from debauchery. His physicians implored him to adopt a lifestyle of temperance in eating and drinking, or he would be dead within a few months

Cornaro became a fanatic about his regimen, subsisting on a daily diet of no more than twelve ounces of solid food and fourteen ounces of wine. He claimed he was never ill again, except once when he gave up the diet. He was notably productive in architecture and civic affairs throughout his long lifetime, constructing four villas, and writing books and articles on many subjects. At eighty-three, he outlined his dietary regimen for longevity in his book *Discorsi della vita sobria* (*Discourse on the Sober Life*), which he rewrote three times by the time he was ninety-five

The Water Trick

Doctors tell us that few people in Western societies drink as much water as they should for optimal health, and many people mistake low-level thirst for low-level hunger. A very helpful tactic for those practicing calorie restriction is to drink a glass of water when first feeling hungry. If you are still hungry twenty minutes later, then maybe it's time to think about eating. Half the time, you were just thirsty, however.

DHEA

DHEA (Dehydroepiandrosterone) is a steroid hormone produced in the adrenal gland and is the most abundant steroid in the bloodstream and found at high levels in brain tissue.

DHEA levels fall 90% from age 20 to age 90. DHEA is known to be a precursor to the numerous steroid sex hormones (including estrogen and testosterone) which serve well-known refunctions. Although the specific mechanisms of action for DHEA are only partially understood, supplemental DHEA has been shown to have anti-aging, anti-obesity and anti-cancer influences.

DHEA levels are directly related to mortality in humans. In a 12-year study of over 240 men aged 50 to 79 years, researchers found that DHEA levels were inversely correlated with mortality, both from heart disease and from all causes. Animal result suggest that supplemental DHEA may prevent disease, reduce mortality, and extend lifespan in humans.

DHEA may also be intimately involved in protecting brain neurons from senility-associated degenera-

tive conditions, like Alzheimer's disease. Not only
do neuronal degenerative conditions occur most
frequently when DHEA levels are lowest, but brain
tissue contains many times more DHEA than is found
in the bloodstream.

Resveratrol

Resveratrol [trans-3,5,4'-trihydroxystilbene] is
found in the skins and seeds of red grapes as well as in
other plants. It is a component of the oriental medicine called Ko-jo-kon and is used to treat diseases of
the blood vessels, heart, and liver. Resveratrol came to
scientific attention at the turn of the century as a possible explanation for the "French Paradox", which is
the low incidence of heart disease among the French
people, who eat a relatively high-fat diet.

Resveratrol is a natural antibiotic produced by
grapes and other plants when under attack by patho-
gens, such as bacteria or fungi. Resveratrol is also nu-
tritional supplement derived from Japanese knotweed
or red grapes. It has been shown to extend the life
span of several short-living species of animals, such as
fruit flies and worms.

In mouse and rat experiments, anti-cancer, anti-
inflammatory, blood-sugar-lowering, chelating and
other beneficial cardiovascular effects of resveratrol
have been reported but not yet replicated in humans.

Resveratrol was reported effective against neuronal
cell dysfunction and cell death, and in theory could
help against diseases such as Huntington's disease and
Alzheimer's disease.

8

LifeStyle

Sandy Shaw and Durk Pearson's book, *Life Extension*, is a comprehensive reference. In 1966, historian Gerald Gruman classified life-extensionists into three main philosophical camps: "meliorists," "incremental-ists," and "immortalists." The meliorists are of the belief that the condition of the aged can be made better, more comfortable, less disease prone, more productive and happier, but that life extension per se either cannot or should not be attempted. Most gerontologists are still of this orientation with the majority of public resources going into the psychology and sociology of aging and into geriatric medicine.

Incrementalists believe that emphasis should be given to developing methods to incrementally increase the life span, which consequently will have the effect of ameliorating the condition of the aged and will give additional time to work on further means toward longevity.

Immortalists believe that most of the effort should be focused on understanding the fundamental causes of aging so that methods can be developed for solving the problem altogether, and eventually the development of non-aging human beings can be achieved.

Exercise

Exercise is the fountain of youth. It encourages growth of new neurons in the brain. When exercise is aerobic and learning a new skill like dancing or playing table tennis – this rejuvenates the brain. Exercise twice a week at a minimum.

Exercise, while not prolonging life, can retard some of the functional declines that accompany aging, such as the loss of muscle **Exercise** mass, capacity for physical effort, flexibility, **is the** endurance, bone strength and efficiency **fountain** of the heart and lungs. It can also help **of youth.** normalize blood pressure, blood sugar and blood cholesterol levels, as well as ward off depression. Exercise does not improve pulmonary function, but increases the amount of oxygen consumption resulting in the reduction of the workload on the heart.

Whole Body Vibration

In whole body vibration the person being treated stands on a vibrating pedestal (the most popular one being the TurboSonic, which gives mechanical oscillations from 3 to 50 Hertz) causing vibrations to be conducted throughout the body to stimulate muscle fibers (myocytes) with three times the strength of gravity. This causes the muscle fibers to contract and relax with greater strength and speed. These powerful muscle contractions enhance muscle strength over a shorter period of time than is feasible with any other form of muscle training. This dramatically enhances flexibility and expedites the recovery of damaged muscles and tendons.

In addition, blood vessels throughout the body are stimulated and circulation is improved. Tendons and ligaments, which are not easily trained, become better toned. The function of intrapelvic muscles and small muscle groups, such as facial muscles, which cannot be strengthened through conventional weight training exercises, are improved. Exercise involving vibration in the vertical direction also causes greater caloric consumption than regular aerobic exercise does.

Whole Body Vibration exercise, in conjunction with conventional muscle exercise, can increase maximum muscle strength by over 30%. It can also reduce the period of training required by 85% and time spent exercising by over 50%. Unlike in conventional muscle training methods involving the lifting of weights, little additional load is imposed on joints, ligaments, and tendons in WBV exercise. Consequently, the risk of exercise-induced injury is reduced to a negligible level.

Research shows that after one vibration training session!, there is a high excretion of Testosterone (+7%) and Growth Hormone (+460%) as well as a drop in the stress hormone cortisol (-32%). This combination has favorable effects on muscle protein synthesis.

Increases in Testosterone and Growth Hormone are important in the functioning of both body and mind. Many complaints of the elderly can be traced to a decrease in these hormones. It is essentially these hormones, together with the female hormone estrogen, which are used to combat geriatric complaints so that it is possible to still enjoy life and vitality even when one has reached old age.

There is nothing worse than experiencing a factory death.

Bone decalcification (osteoporosis) is one of the biggest health problems especially in the elderly and women population. The onset of osteoporosis is partly due to a lack of movement, which causes muscles to gradually weaken, the circulation to diminish and the bones to be inadequately used. As a result of the ageing process, the body produces less hormones such as testosterone, estrogen and growth hormone.

Whole body vibration offers an alternative to vigorous impact exercise: through vibration the muscles automatically become stronger and regain their tone. The circulation improves because the blood vessels in the legs are wide open due to the vibration. At the same time, the pulsation gives a direct stimulus to bone tissue, which in turn stimulates the production of new bone tissue.

Parkinson's disease results from a deficiency in dopamine. Serotonin plays a role in mood, or frame of mind. A shortage of serotonin in the brain can lead to depression. Research shows that vibration training increases the serotonin content in the brain, which may explain why one feels so well after vibration training.

After training, one often sees that the skin of the lower leg is colored pink—a sign that the blood vessels in that area are wide open. In Germany, the effect of vibration training is used as therapy for a disturbed peripheral circulation, particularly in the lower legs, such as in chronic venous insufficiency.

The effect on the muscles is flexively activated via the nervous system. With vibration training, it seems as if pulsations awaken the nerve tract, which could explain the positive effects of vibration training in partial paralysis. In fact, good results have been reported in the experimental treatment of, for example, MS patients.

If you have the bucks you can buy one of these nifty anti-aging, health-promoting machines for your home. Otherwise, they are available at various gyms.

Heat Kills

The higher the normal body temperature of any species the longer will the average life span of its members be, but the lower the average body temperature of an individual member of that species, the greater will that individual's life expectancy be. Body temperature reflects metabolic rate—the amount of food burned per day per unit of body weight. The lower the metabolic rate the greater the life span, and the higher the metabolic rate the shorter the life span.

Heat Stroke

Heat stroke is the most severe form of heat illness and is a life-threatening emergency. It is the result of long, extreme exposure to the sun, in which a person does not sweat enough to lower body temperature. The elderly, infants, persons who work outdoors and those on certain types of medications are most susceptible to heat stroke. It is a condition that develops rapidly and requires immediate medical treatment.

In our quest for life extension, therefore, reduction of our personal metabolic activity rate and our core temperature would seem to be highly desirable objectives.

Although best known for his studies on the anti-aging effects of dietary restriction, Dr. Roy Walford began his career by studying the anti-aging effects of lowering body temperature. As a tribute to his long and productive career, we review these pioneering studies and the singular influence these have had on our own thinking about the potential for lower body temperature to extend the life span of homeotherms.

We show our results from a study of six classical inbred strains of mice that depict marked strain variation in the body temperature response to dietary restriction. In addition, we show a genome scan from a recombinant inbred strain panel in which we identified a significant quantitative trait locus on murine chromosome 9 and a provisional locus on chromosome 17 that specify variation in the response of body temperature to dietary restriction. These discoveries suggest that we can now extend the studies of Dr Walford to critically test whether lower body temperature can prolong the life span of mammals.

Whether slower metabolic processes—which equals lower body temperature and therefore reduced free radical activity—is achieved by dietary restriction—calorie reduction—or by meditation does not seem to matter at all and, as will be made clear in the section on strategies, a combination of both would seem to be highly desirable. Dietary restriction, however, does not always produce a lower metabolic rate—and lower body temperature.

The lower the metabolic rate the greater the life span, and the higher the metabolic rate the shorter the life span.

How to Lower Temperature

First, realize that environmental factors are of secondary importance in altering our core temperature, although there is a clear advantage in them being undemanding. A cold environment calls for both greater metabolic activity and calorie intake with all the negative results that this produces. A pleasantly warm environment, however, reduces metabolic demands and food intake—at least this is true in terms of what is required for heat generation, and is supported by animal studies.

Calorie restriction lowers core temperature, so anyone using this method in a life extension programme would automatically achieve benefits on the hypothermia front as well. There are still other ways of lowering our internal temperature, and these have been employed by Yogis for centuries.

Meditation

The mind can be used to control body temperature. Impressive demonstrations have been given by people using deep relaxation/meditation methods which produced drops of internal temperature of a degree or more.

People wishing to learn to control aspects of body function have for many years used a 'high-tech' version of meditation, biofeedback, to produce effects such as lowered blood pressure, or increased or decreased temperature of body parts—hands made warmer at will where circulation to the limbs is poor, or the head made cooler in response to an impending migraine, are common examples.

Techniques currently widely employed to help induce deep relaxation, and which have highly desirable effects on immune function, such as autogenic training, use visualization of alterations in temperature as part of their methodology, with measurable differences in temperature being evident after only a short time.

Nightly Hibernation

Sleeping is one of the most important things to incorporate into your day if you want to slow down the aging process. Sleep both heals and restores. As you sleep, your body uses energy and resources that would normally be given to more active waking hours to repair your body. When you sleep, cells regenerate, your immune system is restored, and other healing activities take place as you rest. So, if you want to slow down the aging process, make sure to sleep.

Sleep both heals and restores.

Regularly catching only a few hours of sleep can hinder metabolism and hormone production in a way that is similar to the effects of aging and the early stages of diabetes. Chronic sleep loss may speed the onset or increase the severity of age-related conditions such as type 2 diabetes, high blood pressure, obesity, and memory loss.

9

Somatic-Neural-Genetic Preservation

Techniques in this group do not ensure continuous operation of consciousness. They produce reversible metabolic coma. They are alternatives for preserving the structure of tissues until a time of more advanced medical knowledge.

Body "Pickling"

Letting one's body and brain rot seems to imply no possibility at all for your future. Why let the carefully arranged tangle of dendritic growths in your nervous system, which store all your memories get eaten by fungus? Perpetual preservation of your tissues by freezing is available today at moderate cost.

Preservation of Neural Tissue

Those not particularly attached to their bodies can opt for preservation of the essentials: their brains and the instructional codes capable of regrowing something genetically identical to their present bio-machinery.

Biogenetic Methods

Is there any need to experience metabolic coma? We have mentioned ways to gain personal control of the experience, to stave it off by "conventional" longevity techniques, to avoid irreversible dissolution of the systemic substrate. Techniques are now emerging to permit a much more vivid guarantee of personal persistence, a smooth metamorphic transformation into a different form of substrate on which the computer program of consciousness runs.

> Death is a disease waiting to be cured ...When the cure for aging is found, it will not come through faith, prayer, or meditation, but through science—product of the miraculous technowonderland of the modern world.
>
> —SIMON YOUNG
> *Designer Evolution*
> *A Transhumanist Manifesto*

Cellular/DNA Repair

Nanotechnology is the science and engineering of mechanical and electronic systems built to atomic specifications. Nanotechnology has a potential for production of sell-replicating nanomachines living within individual biological cells. These artificial enzymes will effect cellular repair, as damage occurs from mechanical causes, radiation, or other aging effects. Repair of DNA ensures genetic stability.

Store Your DNA

DNA holds information about your biological past, present and future. DNA is your genetic history; the best way to preserve it is by storing your DNA for later analysis.

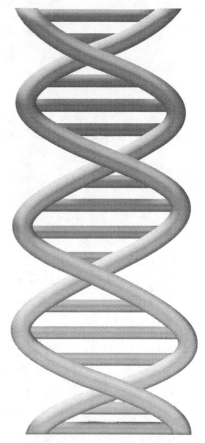

Storing your DNA can help your family in future as genetic testing becomes more affordable, new genes are discovered, and new tests and technologies become available. DNA can be stored at home, in a safe deposit box, or hire a company to store it for you.

DNA is easy to obtain through a quick and painless swabbing of mouth lining. The swab is sent to the DNA company for analysis and storage. Most companies send you a summary DNA analysis card for you to keep.

Stored DNA is an invaluable resource if your family is faced with issues involving identity, relationship, or medical decisions after your death. 0. Solves Social Security issues

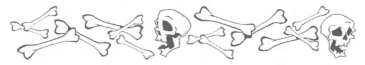

10

ElectRonic Immortality

We can achieve a kind of immortality by leaving behind a trail of archives, biographies, tapes, films, computer files, and publicized noble deeds. The stable knowledge media in our cybernetic society make this a rigorous platform for persistent existence. Knowledge possessed by an individual can be captured in data systems and media.

Personal immortality may still be impossible, but social immortality—continued life in the consciousness and speaking of others—is definitely possible. The cast of characters of our existence survive our death. The survival community is launched at the funeral of the deceased. Even though the dead person has been cremated or buried deep into the ground, his or her spirit lives on in the speech and imagination of the survivors create a kind of spiritual rebirth. Our collective commemoration bestowes a new state of being, a new life—social immortality—onto the decreased person.

The survival community is launched at the funeral of the deceased.

You can accomplish immortality through language. Immortality is life after death. Your name stands for you. Your name is the title of a story—of your life-story. Our role becomes indeed that of "cybers", pilots in our own information ocean.

We remember the life of our public leaders in all fields: our culture heroes. But every family and friendship circle has its own leaders which carry on the tradition: the way we do things together, how to organize our time, what we devote our energy to, what values we hold sacred, what life-style we embody, what celebrations we observe, what spirit we adore and serve.

— DR. ROLF VON ECKARTSBERG

Today much of the wisdom of personal life seems to get lost when the person dies. Dr. Rolf Von Eckartsberg encourages us to revision.

Author Your Life

Many people use a video to make a last will and testament to leave instructions for how possessions are to be distributed. Through the act of making your re-vision you reach beyond your death to affect the future.

Writings you have authored, and art-works or knowledge-works you have created achieve a kind of immortality as creative mini life-sums in the listener's or reader's consciousness and discourse. Your work moves beyond your control into immortality. Even during your life-time becomes a voice on a CD that repeats in new encounters with newcomers, or waits on the shelves of libraries or in electro-magnetic storage to be played.

What we have done for ourselves alone
dies with us; what we have done for
others and the world remains and is im-
mortal.

—ALBERT PIKE

We are reborn through language in the remem-
brance of the heirs and the surviving community,
through the circulation of life stories and life portraits.

Immortality Portfolio

Gather photographs and mementos that embody
significant events and relationships in your life. Record the inner and outer events of
your life in a journal. Collect stories that weave the images and mementos into the meaningful fabric of
your life into your "immortality port-
folio" to be preserved on a CD. Von Eckartsberg views
this as a kind of existential time-capsule.

**Your work moves
beyond your
control into
immortality.**

Everybody is a super-star in his or her
own ensemble, an irreplaceable valued
person. Every person's life can be considered to be a work of art, worthy of
appreciation.

— DR. ROLF VON ECKARTSBERG

After you have gathered your immortality materi-
als, write a script to narrate your creative production.

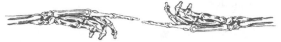

Life-Sum-Video

Retirement is a good time for personal reminiscing, life-sum constructions and co-creative personal video-production. Create an electronic immortality portfolio that contains all the records of your life—written, photographed, filmed, spoken or videotaped.

Fashion a story-line from your total life-collage. Integrate events, relationships, projects, achievements and failures, glories and defeats, joys and sorrows into a bio-narrative. Doing such a life-summing can be difficult.

Electronic Wakes

Life-sums and immortality portfolios can be shared with family and friends at "electronic wakes" and in "electronic cemeteries and memorials" and even in "immortality communication satellites" and available for viewing at anniversaries to commemorate you.

Personality Data-Base Transmission

"Head Coach", developed by Futique, Inc., is a psychoactive computer software. The program allows the user—performer—to digitize and store thoughts on a routine daily basis. If you leave, let us say, twenty years of daily computer-stored records of thought-performance, your grandchildren, a century down the line, can "know" and replay your information habits and mental performances. They will be able to "share and relive experiences" in considerable detail. To take

a mundane example, if you moves in a chess game are
stored, your descendants can relive, move by move, a
game played by Great-Great-Grandmother in the past
century.

The program allows hackers to write their own
movie using Gibson's characters and setting. They can
check their talents later against Hollywood's version
of *Neuromancer*.

As passive reading is replaced by "active rewrit-
ing," later generations will be able to relive how we
performed the great stories of our time.

Yet more intriguing is the possibility of implement-
ing the knowledge extracted over time from a person:
their beliefs, preferences, and tendencies, as a set of
algorithms guiding a program capable of acting in
a manner functionally identical to the person. Ad-
vances in robotics technology will take these "Turing
creatures" away from being mere "brains in bottles"
to hybrids capable of interacting sensorily with the
physical world.

If you want to immortalize
your consciousness—
record and digitize.

11

BRain-CompuTeR TRansFeR

When a computer becomes obsolete, we don't discard the data it contains. The hardware is merely a temporary vehicle of implementation for structures of information. We transfer the data to new systems for continued use. Decreasing costs of computer storage and WORM memory systems mean that no information generated today ever need be lost.

We can consider building an artificial computational substrate both functionally and structurally identical to the brain—and perhaps the body—of a person. This can be achieved with predicted future capabilities of nanotechnology. Communicating nanomachines that pervade the organism may analyze the neural and cellular structure and transfer the information obtained to machinery capable of growing, atom by atom, an identical copy.

> Soul is the animating and vital principle in man credited with the faculties of thought, action, and emotion, and conceived as forming an immaterial entity distinguishable from but temporarily coexistent with his body.
>
> *American Heritage Dictionary*

From the perspective of information theory, "immaterial" can be understood as "invisible to the naked eye, i.e., atomic-molecular-electronic," and "soul" refers to information processed and stored in microscopic-cellular, molecular, atomic packages. "Soul" becomes any information that "lives," i.e., that is capable of being retrieved and communicated

Preserve Your Signal Capacity

All tests for "death" at every level of measurement—nuclear, neural, bodily, galactic—involve signal unresponsiveness. From this viewpoint, the immortality options become cybernetic methods of preserving one's unique signal capacity. There are as many souls as there are ways of storing and communicating data. Tribal lore defines the racial soul. The DNA is a molecular soul. The brain is a neurological soul. Electron storage creates the silicon soul. Nanotechnology makes possible the atomic soul.

Kon-Tiki of the Flesh

What we taken for granted as the perishable human creature, in the not to distant future, will be a mere historical curiosity, one point amidst unimaginable, multidimensional diversity of form. Individuals, or groups of adventurers, will be free to choose to reassume flesh-and-blood form, constructed for the occasion by the appropriate science.

> Preserve your body -
> Preserve your brain-
> Preserve your DNA.
>
> To immortalize: digitize!

Mind Uploading

If the neural network of the brain can be thought of as hardware, then the human mind is the software running on it. Mind uploading is transferring this "software" from the hardware of the human brain to another processing environment, such as a robot or quantum computer.

No technology exists yet to upload your mind. It is still a speculative process, but as we've long been told: "Whatever the mind can conceive and believe, the mind can achieve." Since it's pretty easy to "conceive" consciousness uploading, we can count on it to be developed sometime soon.

Most theoretical approaches to mind uploading are based on the idea of recreating or simulating the underlying neural network. This approach would theoretically eliminate the need to understand how such a system works if the component neurons and their connections can be simulated with enough accuracy.

When the mind is transferred into a computer, the subject would become a form of artificial intelligence, sometimes called an *infomorph* or *noömorph*. When the mind upload is transferred into an artificial body, to which its consciousness is confined, the resulting being is a robot.

When uploading, the physical human brain does not move into a new robotic shell; rather, consciousness is recorded and/or transferred to a new robotic brain, which generates responses indistinguishable from the original organic brain.

Once an individual is moved to virtual simulation, the only input needed would be energy, which would be provided by large computing device hosting those minds. All the food, drink, moving, travel, and so forth would just need energy to provide those computations.

Why Become An Upload?

Nick Bostrom of the Philosophy Department of Oxford University has analyzed the advantages of being an upload. Uploads would not be subject to biological aging and would continue so long as the replication and all of its copies are preserved. The risk of damage can be covered for by back-up copies of uploads regularly so that you can be re-booted if something bad does happen. Besides existing far beyond a human lifespan, you can "live" very economically because uploads don't need food or housing, or clothing either.

When you run on a fast computer, you can think vastly faster than when in human form. Among other benefits, you experience more subjective time because reality around moves at such a slower pace than you think, so you live more, during any given day. Another fabulous benefit is that you would be able to travel at the speed of light as an information pattern. You could be on the beach in Hawaii one minute, then in an instant you can be hiking in the snow in the Swiss Alps! Being able to travel at the speed of light would be essential in the future after Space is colonized. You will be able to leap galaxies in a single second—perhaps faster.

Uploads of narcissists and megalomaniacs might become problematic because uploads don't have to find a "lover" to reproduce. All they have to do is to save a duplication. And they could duplicate themselves infinitely.

Scientists, thinkers and intelligent people would be uploaded and moved to a virtual environment when they die. In this virtual environment, their brain capacity would be expanded by speed and storage of quantum computers. These creative geniuses would continue making innovations to be sent to the human world and technological development would speed up.

Cyborging

Some envision replacing brain neurons one at a time while keeping consciousness intact, which is process known as *cyborging*.

The first step is to map the brain. Then it is replaced piece-by-piece with computer devices that perform the same function as the brain regions replaced. Then the patient is brought back to consciousness to validate that his or her subjective experience of reality continues unchanged.

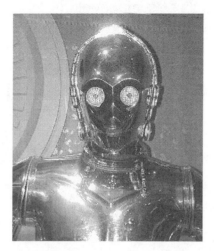

Next, the patient's brain is re-mapped and another piece is replaced, and the procedure repeated until, the patient exists on a purely hardware medium and can be safely extricated from the physical body.

Transhumanism

The quest for immortality is one of the most ancient and deep-rooted of human aspirations. It has been an important theme in human literature from the very earliest preserved written story, The Epic of Gilgamesh, and in innumerable narratives and myths ever since. It underlies the teachings of world religions about spiritual immortality and the hope of an afterlife. If death is part of the natural order, so too is the human desire to overcome death.

Before transhumanism, the only hope of evading death was through reincarnation or otherworldly resurrection. Those who viewed such religious doctrines as figments of our own imagination had no alternative but to accept death as an inevitable fact of our existence. Secular worldviews, including traditional humanism, would typically include some sort of explanation of why death was not such a bad thing after all. Some existentialists even went so far as to maintain that death was necessary to give life meaning!

That people should make excuses for death is understandable. Until recently there was absolutely nothing anybody could do about it, and it made some degree of sense then to create comforting philosophies according to which dying of old age is a fine thing ("deathism"). If such beliefs were once relatively harmless, and perhaps even provided some therapeutic benefit, they have now outlived their purpose. Today, we can foresee the possibility of eventually abolishing aging and we have the option of taking active measures to stay alive until then, through life extension techniques and, as a last resort, cryonics. This makes the illusions of deathist philosophies dangerous, indeed fatal, since they teach helplessness and encourage passivity.

Posthuman

Uploads and other future beings whose basic capacities radically exceed those of humans can no longer be considered "human" by our current definitions of human. These future beings—which may not have any physical form—are called *posthumans*. Transhumans are an intermediary form between the human and the posthuman.

As we evolve into posthumans nanotechnology will redesign the human vehicle using genetic engineering, psychopharmacology, anti-aging therapies, neural interfaces, advanced information management tools, memory enhancing drugs, wearable computers, cognitive metaprogramming and other advanced technologies.

Posthuman Lifestyle

We can hardly imagine what reality and living will be a posthuman person. Posthumans will have experiences and concerns that we cannot fathom. Not only will their minds be more powerful than ours but they will employ different cognitive architectures and new sensory modalities. They will live in virtual realities rather than as beings on earth. The boundaries between posthuman minds will not be as sharply defined. Posthuman minds will share memories and experiences directly, rather than through the cumbersome talking and writing methods that humans use to communicate with each other.

Singularity

There will be a point in the future when the rate of technological development becomes so rapid that the progress-curve becomes nearly vertical and within a very brief time, the world might be transformed almost beyond recognition. This hypothetical point is referred to as *the singularity*. The creation of a rapidly self-enhancing greater-than-human intelligence is the probably pre-requisite cause of a singularity.

Enhancing intelligence will, in this scenario, at some point lead to a positive feedback loop: smarter systems can design systems that are even more intelligent, and can do so more swiftly than the original human designers. This positive feedback effect would be powerful enough to drive an intelligence explosion that could quickly lead to the emergence of a superintelligent system of surpassing abilities.

A superintelligent intellect—a superintelligence, sometimes called "ultraintelligence"—can radically outperform the best human brains in practically every field, including scientific creativity, general wisdom, and social skills. Strong superintelligence refers to an intellect that is not only faster than

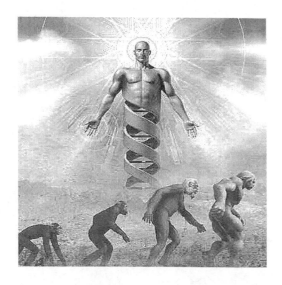

a human brain but also smarter in a qualitative sense—
meaning a kind of quantum leap to a meta-intelligence.

Viral Existence
in the Matrix

The previous option permitted personal survival through isomorphic mapping of neural structure
to silicon—or some other arbitrary medium of implementation. It also suggests the possibility of survival
as an entity in what amounts to a reification of Jung's
collective unconscious: the global information network.

In the 21st Century imagined by novelist William
Gibson, wily cybernauts will not only store themselves
electronically, but do so in the form of a "computer
virus," capable of traversing computer networks and of
self-replication as a guard against accidental or mali-
cious erasure by others or other programs.

Given the ease of copying computer-stored information, one could exist simultaneously in many forms.
Where the "I" is in this situation is a matter for philosophy. We believe that consciousness would persist in
each form, running independently—and ignorant of
each other's self-manifestation unless in communication with it—and cloned at each branch point.

Note: The above options for voluntary reversible metabolic coma and auto-metamorphosis are not
mutually exclusive. The intelligent person needs little
encouragement to explore all these possibilities, and
to design many new other alternatives to going belly-
up in line with management

12

Re-Creational Reprogramming

The nervous system consists of eight potential circuits, or "gears," or mini-brains. These eight stages of intelligence are biological, emotional, mental-symbolic, social, aesthetic, neurological-cybernetic, genetic, atomic-nanotech. Four of these brains are in the usually active left lobe and concerned with terrestrial survival. The other four are extraterrestrial, residing in the "silent" or inactive right lobe to be used for future evolution.

At each of these stages there is an input recognition stage, followed by a programming-reprogramming stage, and an output communication stage.

Conscious-Intelligence Levels

At our present crude and primitive level of understanding it is appropriate to consider eight levels of consciousness-intelligence.

1. THE BIO-SURVIVAL CIRCUIT: The autonomic nervous-system that mediates physiological satisfactions and warnings; pain-somatic-pleasure;

2. THE EMOTIONAL CIRCUIT: The mid-brain that mediates mammalian emotion, aggression, territorial instincts, power, security;

3. THE DEXTERITY-SYMBOLISM CIRCUIT: The left-brain or dominant hemisphere that mediates thinking, manual dexterity, language, symbolic learning, manufacture;

4. THE SOCIAL-SEXUAL CIRCUIT: The domestication-socialization circuits that mediate cultural behavior, sex-role-impersonation, moral-ethical behavior necessary for acceptance by society;

5. THE NEUROSOMATIC CIRCUIT: The right-brain and sensory-somatic circuits that mediate awareness of body-function, rhythm, pattern, erotic-hedonic, aesthetic behavior;

6. THE NEUROELECTRIC CIRCUIT: The meta-programming circuits that allow consciousness of the brain as a bio-electric loom, fabricating realities;

7. THE NEUROGENETIC CIRCUIT: The neurogenetic circuits that allow consciousness of Brain-RNA-DNA communication and direct deciphering of genetic blueprint;

8. THE NEURO-ATOMIC CIRCUIT: The frontal-lobe circuits that permit direct awareness of and communication with electronic-atomic information, such as brain-computer linkups.

These levels are listed in order of the age, speed, power, complexity, expansiveness, and planful wisdom of the energy structure.

Re-Creational Programming

To reprogram, we must activate the circuits in the brain, which mediate that particular dimension of intelligence. Once this circuit is "turned on," we can reimprint or reprogram.

Cognitive neurology suggests that the most direct way to reprogram emotional responses is to reactivate the emotional stage and reprogram, replace fear with laughter. To reprogram sexual responses, it is logical to reactivate and re-experience the original teenage imprints and to re-imprint and to re-imprint new erotic stimuli and new sexual responses.

The seventh circuit is most relevant to our discussion here. It kicks in when the nervous system receives signals from the DNA-RNA dialogue. Hindu and Sufis adepts, who are advanced at this level, spoke of past lives, reincarnation and immortality and foresaw evolution aeons before Darwin.

Other metaphors for this circuit include Theosophy's akashic records of Theosophy, Jung's collective unconscious, and Grof and Ring's phylogenetic unconscious. The visions of past and future evolution reported by those who have near-death experiences describe the trans-time seventh circuit.

Entheogens, like peyote and LSD, are the seventh circuit neurotransmitter. The Seventh Circuit VII opens the genetic archives activated by anti-histone proteins. The DNA memory coiling back to the dawn of life. The evolutionary function of the seventh circuit and its evolutionary, aeon-spanning tunnel-reality is to prepare us for conscious immortality and interspecies symbiosis.

One great thing about being old and "senile"—it liberates you from social games. People *expect* old folks to be crotchety, to break taboo boundaries in social behavior by blurting out honest home-truths, particularly when no suffering fools gladly. In fact, realizing this, the old person often turns sly trickster, taking advantage of the opportunity to have a "second childhood," or in other words another crack at crazy wisdom. All old people have an opportunity to play "rascal guru."

—TIMOTHY LEARY
Design for Dying

Develop New Rituals

Our cultural taboos have prohibited the development of much detailed work in this area, but some important research has been done by E. J. Gold described in The New American Book of the Dead. We need new rituals to guide the post-body transition.

Dying is a difficult process, with many fears and anxieties, yet mysterious and wondrous. It involves the body and the soul in the greatest transition we will ever make.

Rituals help heal the pain of letting go, offering reconciliation and peace, while at the same time connecting with the living. End-of-life rituals help a person die a peaceful and sacred death.

Pre-Incarnation Exercises

Use your preferred altered-state method—drugs,
hypnosis, shamanic trance, voodoo ritual, born-again
frenzies—to create future scripts for yourself.

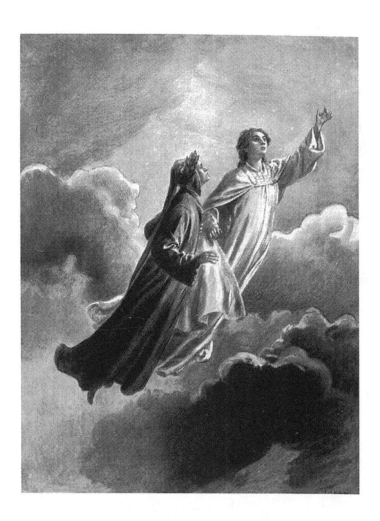

13

mummification

In the 1970s Summum introduced "Modern Mummification," a form of mummification that Summum claims uses modern techniques along with aspects of ancient methods. The company's mummification process preserves the body as a means to aid the essence as it transitions to a new destination. Summum calls this "transference," and the concept seems to correlate with ancient Egyptian reasons for mummification. Today, Summum is the only organization in the world to offer this remarkable and distinguished tradition.

Summum uses a chemical process that maintains the body's natural look. The process requires that the body stay submerged in a tank of preservation fluid for several months. Summum claims its process preserves the body so well that the DNA will remain intact far into the future, leaving open the possibility for cloning when the process is perfected for humans.

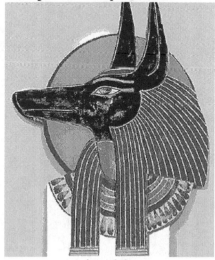

Anubis

Summum recommends your Mummiform be enshrined in a sanctuary/mausoleum or cemetery space that maintains a moderate temperature of 72° F (22° C)so that your mummy doesn't freeze or get too warm.

Mummification

The traditional mummification process has two stages. The first one is called embalming. The embalming process cleans the body for the wrapping, the second stage. The wrapping has a number of special steps.

Embalming

First, the body is washed with palm wine and rinsed with water from the Nile River. A small cut is made in the left side of the body and the liver, lungs, small intestines, and large intestines, are removed. Next the brains are removed. The Egyptians used a long hook inserted through the nose to pull the brains out.

The body is covered and stuffed with natron. This is known as the drying stage, which is forty days. Then the body is washed with water from the Nile River and covered with sweet smelling oils. Finally, the body is stuffed with dry things, such as sawdust, leaves, and linen and covered with more oils. The internal organs are put into the canopic jars.

Wrapping

The head and neck are wrapped. Then fingers and toes are wrapped, followed by wrapping the arms and legs. Sacred amulets are placed.

The spells from the book of the dead are read. The arms and legs are tied together. A scroll is placed between the hands of the deceased. The full body is wrapped and is painted with liquid resin as glue. A cloth with Osiris painted on it is wrapped around the body. Linen stripes are wrapped around the body to hold the cloth in place.

The mummy is put in the first coffin. The mummy is put in the second coffin. The funeral is held. The opening of the mouth ceremony is performed. The mummy is put in the sarcophagus. The mummy is put in its final resting place, the tomb.

Anubis

Anubis is the god of embalming and the dead. He was believed to watch over the process of mummification

Mummify Yourself

There are two dozen mummified Japanese monks known as Sokushinbutsu. For three years the priests eat a special diet consisting of nuts and seeds, while undergoing rigorous physical activity to stripped them of body fat. Then they eat only bark and roots for another three years and drink a poisonous tea made from the sap of the Urushi tree, which contains Urushiol—same stuff that makes poison ivy—used to lacquer bowls. This caused vomiting and a rapid loss of bodily fluids.

Finally, the self-mummifying monk locks himself in a stone tomb barely larger than his body, where he stays in the lotus position. His only connection to the outside world is an air tube and a bell. Each day he rings a bell to let those outside know that he is still alive. When the bell stops ringing, the tube is removed and the tomb sealed.

Self-mummification is a long and extremely painful process that requires a mastery of self-control and denial of physical sensation. Not all monks who attempt self-mummification succeed, but the pay-off for the ones who do so is quite high. They were raised to the status of Budda, put on display, and tended to by their followers.

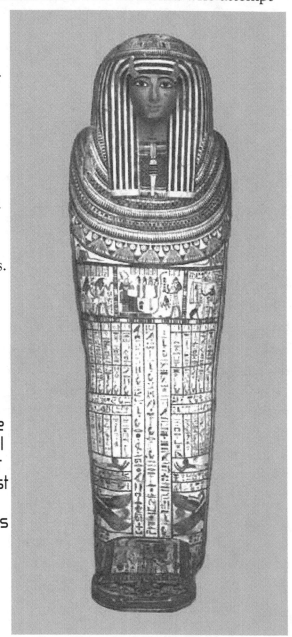

If you are mummified you must be very special indeed. For only the most valued are preserved as mummies.

14

Voluntary Dying

Officials who wish to control the mortem process called suicide. Traditionally, self-induced death has been considered a cowardly or insane attempt to interfere with the natural order. Those who wished to manage and direct their own dying were condemned by law and custom.

In a pagan or nature-attuned tribal culture, there is a common-sense genetic wisdom implied in this passive acceptance of one's termination. The brain continually monitors the vital functions of the body, and as the body starts failing, terminal programs take over. The brain quietly shuts down the body and during the few minutes between body death and neurological death, the brain's hundred billion neurons probably enjoy an astonishing "timeless" review of all and everything.

In the late 20th Century, however, mechanical medical science started "interfering" quite dramatically with the "natural" order. Tubes and machines are now used to keep patients "alive" long after the cessation of consciousness. A stroke victim who twenty years ago might have died in an hour can now be revived, only to spend years in machine-induced coma.

Most people are shocked and outraged by mechanical-medical methods that strip dignity and human consciousness from the terminal-coma patient. The American Medical Association has supported the right of the family to remove medical treatment from terminally ill comatose patients.

Then there is the problem of intractable pain suffered by patients terminally ill from "artificial" diseases caused by industrial pollution like cancer, which cause agonizing pain. The brain housed in the body of a person living in the industrial low-rent, tacky culture of the late 20th Century is not programmed to handle these new diseases. The brain is capable of producing endorphin pain-killers naturally. The brain is beautifully geared to slowly, gracefully turn out the lights for humans—as they do for other animals. Our sisters and brothers, the other pack animals like wolves and dogs and cats, for example, manage to die in dignity without screaming to veterinarians for sedation or priests for extreme unction.

But the factory-hospital environment, run efficiently by factory managers—doctors and nurses, is a very strange environment for any normal hundred-billion-neuron brain. Hospitalized patients whose brains are imprinted to perform as factory units when terminally ill and in great pain passionately beg to be put out of their hopeless misery.

Quality of Life

Quality of life is a measure the degree of well-being we feel. It is not something tangible like how much cash you have in the bank. There are two components to quality of life. Health, home, and money contribute to physical comfort whereas emotional well-being makes up the psychological component.

Quality of life is subjective to each individual. We can't determine it from across the room—it's internal to each individual. However, we can make generalizations. Obviously diet, shelter, safety, needs must be at least minimally met. Also vital relationships, opportunities for creativity, as well as freedoms and rights.

Evaluating your quality of life is the first step in death designing. If you are suffering from a painful condition with little hope of improvement, life can feel like a torture rather than a pleasure. Losing one's mental faculties can reduce one to a child-like dependent state. The Quality of Life Inventory can help you to explore variables contributing to or detracting from your quality of life.

Quality of Life Inventory

Senility Score Board

I. Physical

Health

Mobility

Vitality

Physical Attractiveness

Dexterity

Physical Strength

II. Psychological
Mental Ability
Interpersonal Relationships
Self Confidence
Enthusiasm – Life Spirit

III. Social
Social Sophistication
Environment
Financial Security

Dying is the single most important thing you will do your entire life. My existence and work was guided by these basic principles: Maintain a sense of humour. Think for yourself. Question authority. Love and celebrate chaotics. Follow the Laws of Levities—lighten up. Do it with friends because increasing illumination and understanding is a team sport

Design Your Own Death
Fundamentalist religious groups and neo-feudal officials oppose any "pro-choice" initiative that allows individuals to manage their own lives. These groups also are actively opposed to "euthanasia."

Improving health means increasing the quality of life not just avoiding death

—PATCH ADAMS

By the end of the 20th Century, a growing movement had developed in California to allow terminally ill patients to arrange for their own dying: Americans Against Human Suffering (Freedom of Choice for Physician Aid-in Dying). In Holland, "euthanasia on request" is made available after a prudent, suitable period of review. Since 1992, Michigan doctor Jack Kevorkian has repeatedly tested the law by helping his terminally ill patients exercise their right to choose the time and manner of their death.

Dr. Death

Jack Kevorkian was the greatest taboo smasher of all when he made control over one's own death a national issue. Imagine the state forcing us to stay alive when we're suffering intensely and have make a considered decision to move on. That's *torture!* He took revolutionary action for the rights of the dying—those experiencing suffering as the result of the extended dying process—to choose our personal time and method of "passing on".

Kevorkian "pushed the envelop" far beyond what the right to die societies in America were at the time working for— assistance in dying only for the advanced terminally ill. "Dr. Death" as the media dubbed him, helped people with painful terminal illnesses plus people with degenerative diseases.

Andy Rooney, the long-time purveyor of droll comment at the end of the television news show *60 Minutes* interviewed Kevorkian in 1996, when there was this exchange....

Rooney: "I think the American public is puzzled by you. They don't know whether you're a medical philosopher or a nut. Which are you?

Kevorkian: "Probably both. You might say I'm a philosophic nut, or a nutty philosopher. It doesn't matter. Words don't mean anything. If you dig into anybody's character you can find eccentricities you can characterize as nutty."

Sentencing him to 10- 25 years in prison, Judge Jessica Cooper said, "This trial was not about the political and mortal correctness of euthanasia. It was about you, sir. It was about lawlessness. You had the audacity to go on national television, show the world what you did and dare the legal system to stop you. Well, sir, consider yourself stopped."

—DEREK HUMPHRY
The Good Euthanasia Guide
Where, What and Who in Choices in Dying

15

CLONING

Biologically based replication of genetically identical personal copies of yourself, at any time desired, is approaching the possible. Sex is fun, but sexual reproduction is biologically inefficient, suited mainly for inducing genetic variation in species that still advance through the accidents of luck in random combination. The idea is to reserve sex as a means of communication and to reproduce asexually!

Some silicon visionaries believe that natural evolution of the human species—or at least their branch of it —is near completion. They are no longer interested in merely procreating, but in designing their successors. Carnegie-Mellon robotics scientist Hans Moravec writes,

We owe our existence to organic evolution. But we owe it little loyalty. We are on the threshold of a change in the universe comparable to the transition from nonlife to life.

Human society has now reached a turning point in the operation of the process of evolution at which the next evolutionary step of the species is under our control. Or, more correctly, the next steps, occurring in parallel, and resulting in an explosion of diversity of the human species. We are no longer dependent on fitness in any physical sense for survival. Our quantum appliances and older mechanical devices provide the requisite means in all circumstances. In the near future, the merging methods of computer and biological technology will make the human form a matter totally determined by individual choice.

As a flesh-and-blood species we are moribund, stuck at "a local optimum," to borrow a term from mathematical optimization theory. Beyond this horizon, which humankind has reached, lies the unknown, the scarcely imagined. We will design our children, and co-evolve intentionally with the cultural artifacts that are our progeny.

Humans already come in some variety of races and sizes. In comparison to what 'human" will mean within the next century, we humans are at present as indistinguishable from one another as are hydrogen molecules. Our anthropocentrism will decrease.

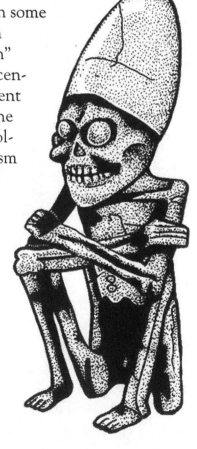

Consider two principle categorizations of the form of the human of the future, one more biological-like: a bio/machine hybrid of any desired form; and one not biological at all: an "electronic life" on the computer networks. Human as machine, and human *in* machine.

Human as machine is perhaps more easily conceived. We already have crude prosthetic implants, artificial limbs, valves, and entire organs. The continuing improvements in the old-style mechanical technology slowly increase the thoroughness of human-machine integration.

Human beings are not "souls" or "spirits" but evolved, biological beings genetically programmed to survive, reproduce, and self-destruct.

—SIMON YOUNG
Designer Evolution
A Transhumanist Manifesto

The electronic life form of human in machine is even more alien to our current conceptions of humanity. Through storage of one's belief systems as on-line data structures, driven by selected control structures (the electronic analog to will?), one's neuronal apparatus will operate in silicon as it did on the wetware of the brain, although faster, more accurately, more self-mutably, and, if desired, immortally.

16

PRE-MORTEM HIBERNATION

This planful procedure takes on a different meaning when the person does not "die," but slides into cryonic or brain-bank hibernation. This option is called "pre-mortem suspension." It was ruled legal in California, in a case brought by the Alcor Foundation.

The Alcor Life Extension Foundation is the world leader in cryonics, cryonics research, and cryonics technology. Cryonics is the science of using ultra-cold temperature to preserve human life with the intent of restoring good health when technology becomes available to do so. Alcor is a non-profit organization located in Scottsdale, Arizona, founded in 1972.

What is Cryonics?

Cryonics is a speculative life support technology that seeks to preserve human life in a state that will be viable and treatable by future medicine. It is expected that future medicine will include mature nanotechnology, and the ability to heal at the cellular and molecular levels.

Cryonics is the speculative practice of using cold to preserve the life of a person who can no longer be supported by ordinary medicine. The goal is to carry the person forward through time.

Cryonics is the speculative practice of using cold to preserve the life of a person who can no longer be supported by ordinary medicine. The goal is to carry the person forward through time, for however many decades or centuries might be necessary, until the preservation process can be reversed, and the person restored to full health.

Three little know facts:

1) Life can be stopped and restarted if its basic structure is preserved.

Human embryos are routinely preserved for years at temperatures that completely stop the chemistry of life. Adult humans have survived cooling to temperatures that stop the heart, brain, and all other organs from functioning for up to an hour. These and many other lessons of biology teach us that life is a particular structure of matter. Life can be stopped and restarted if cell structure and chemistry are preserved sufficiently well.

2) Vitrification (not freezing) can preserve biological structure very well.

Adding high concentrations of chemicals called cryoprotectants to cells permits tissue to be cooled to very low temperatures with little or no ice formation. The state of no ice formation at temperatures below -120°C is called vitrification. It is now possible to physically vitrify organs as large as the human brain, achieving excellent structural preservation without freezing.

3) Methods for repairing structure at the molecular level can now be foreseen.

The emerging science of nanotechnology will eventually lead to devices capable of extensive tissue repair and regeneration, including repair of individual cells one molecule at a time. This future nanomedicine could theoretically recover any preserved person in which the basic brain structures encoding memory and personality remain intact.

What this means is, *if* survival of structure means survival of the person; *if* cold can preserve essential structure with sufficient fidelity; *if* foreseeable technology can repair injuries of the preservation process; *then* cryonics should work, even though it cannot be demonstrated to work today.

The object of cryonics is to prevent death by preserving sufficient cell structure and chemistry so that recovery (including recovery of memory and personality) remains possible by foreseeable technology. If indeed cryonics patients are recoverable in the future, then clearly they were never really dead in the first place. Today's physicians will simply have been wrong about when death occurs, as they have been so many times in the past. The argument that cryonics cannot work because cryonics patients are dead is a circular argument.

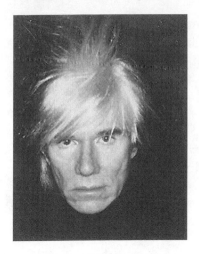

Hibernating Andy

Andy Warhol, the modern artist, became interested in cryonic immortality—as he so quaintly called it—when he learned that Walt Disney's soul—brain—and flesh is being hibernetically frozen and preserved until Eric Drexier's M.I.T. nanotechnology—atom stacking—has mastered the logical steps to re-animate and restore him—i.e., Walt Disney.

Andy shared the almost universal belief that Walt Disney was one of the most important members of the 20th Century. You see, Walt Disney created "screen-iconic" entities of such global-mythic attraction that they are immediately recognized and loved by almost every quark on this globe. Andy told me over and over again that Walt Disney created pop culture. By pop, Andy means the popularization, humanization of ideas.

Andy was well aware of my assignment as publicity director of the Alcor Foundation to personalize, popularize, humanize, Disneyize the cryonic-hibernation re-animation option. And neither did he!

The Legal Authorization

The first logical question in anyone's mind is: Did Andy choose neurological (head-soul) freezing? Or total body cryonic hibernation?

At first he was undecided. Andy could, of course, afford total body ($100,000), but he seemed more interested in the neurological option ($35,000). Andy liked the idea that, when his meat functions flat-lined, his brain—soul—could be preserved, awaiting the kinky moment when an attractive young person of either or both sexes would—as the tragic result of some car accident after the Junior Prom or a crack-house shoot-out—be lying comatose in the emergency ward, a brain-dead neo-mort, available for a transplant from a super-attractive brain.

I promised Andy, on three occasions, that I would do everything necessary to prevent him from being buried by the MOMA or the equally insidious Valerie Solanis/Saint Patrick Cathedral gang, or turned over to the M&O—maggot and oven—crowd, i.e., destroyed by legally sanctioned DNA-killers. In return for this promise, Andy gave me his power of eternity, which I transmitted by American Express.

On these three occasions, Andy begged me, "Please don't let my body be exhibited publicly in the Museum of Modern Art or Saint Patrick's Cathedral."

There is no greater gift of charity you can give than helping a person to die well.

—SOGYAL RINPOCHE
The Tibetan Book of Living and Dying

The documents signed by Andy authorizing his hi-bernation-re-animation have been properly affidavit-ted. Andy's plans will remain, as per his wishes, secret.

There were several witnesses: Ultra Violet, who still wants to rock 'n' roll like days of old despite the fact that she's become a Mormon or a Christian Scientist. I have witnesses! Viva, two. These were two, fine pioneer women that Andy signed up in his weirdo wagon train. Edie Sedgwick, three. Andy, by the way, recorded these conversations and shot Polaroid pix of all present.

Dying is the most embarrassing thing that can ever happen to you, because someone's got to take care of all your details.

—ANDY WARHOL

After Andy Deanimated

Andy wrote about death: "I don't believe in it, because you're not around to know that it's happened. I can't say anything about it because I'm not prepared for it."

Okay. Let's get organized here.

I am on American Airlines flight 103 from J. Fitz. K. to Miami, Florida, my flop-top computer lapping-flapping away, writing to the Alcor Foundation to report on how the cryonic suspension—hibernation—of Andy Warhol's body and soul was accomplished.

At 6:00 A.M. PST on Hybernation-Day-minus-1, I was notified that Andy's meat vehicle was deteriorating sharply and that cardiac arrest was, at most, two days away. I reserved space on the noon flight to New York. My cover for this mission was to model a Guess gene commercial shoot by Helmut Newton.

My true mission was:

1. To assist in the removal of Andy's body from the hospital to our mortuary on West 91st Street;

2. To assist in the cryonic freezing of Andy;

3. To ship the cryonic patient—Andy—to the California depository;

4. To attend the Andy Warhol funeral at Saint Patrick's Cathedral and the subsequent ghoulish body-destruction festivities to see if there were any signs that anyone was aware that Andy's body had been liberated from Christian neuro-terrorists who were so enthusiastically driven to consign all of Warhol's organic tissue-information banks to the ever-hungry worms. My flight was delayed; so I called Grace Jones from the airport to tell her I'd be late.

Grace was not part of the freezing operation, although she played major roles in some of Andy's last public triumphs. Andy symbolically married Grace in public shortly before his hibernation. His very last video performance occurred on Grace's MTV production of "I'm Not Perfect, Nut I'm Perfect for You." Andy, a Cabalist and numerologist, knew at the time that his nights were numbered.

I suggest you play this MTV tape and observe Andy's comatic state. How well he concealed his 1968 illness!

Andy's chronic impression was contagious. It nibbled at my brain like worms. These are certainly strange daze!

Even if you've lived your life like a complete slob, you can die with terrific style.

—TIMOTHY LEARY
Design for Dying

Writing become difficulty, and I have to be careful not to let my imagery become too disteanciated. My writing is nothing if not the history of my illness. The entire staff of *Interview* magazine is in danger of suffering from the same chronic impression.

The role of the Museum of Modern Art in the matter I not exemplary. They showed no great enthusiasm for Andy during his long, long period of dying (1968-1987). And then they go after him *con brio* as soon as they think—erroneously— that he is dead. The bake-meats are barely frozen cold upon the funeral table when MOMA announces the palladium of a full-scale retrospective!

Well, the joke's on they who are marketing Andy like a combination of Jesus Christ and Donald Duck, and don't realize that Andy is not dead, but sleeping. Next to... guess who?

$3,500 Phone Bill Aloft

I was, at this point in time, 35,000 feet high, a nervous wreck, suffering mental fatigue with the portable phone linked to my laptop, jacking into certain counterculture sectors of cyberspace, of which there are literally infinite numbers. I was not phoning my bookmaker, undertaker, pimp, wall-street pallbearer. I was not ordering call girls or fast pizza delivery.

I spent a most pleasant hour on "interscreen" digitizing with the Chaos Hacker group in Germany, who are very well known to Interpol and the KGB. We have developed these hilarious, international, digital intersex romances. I tell you, you can learn a lot about human nature quarking around in Cyberia! Digital intercourse is the best way to prepare for the juicy, sweaty, warm-flash transaction of "hard reality."

At last, my touchdown in Eastern Metropolis! Am I happy? No way! My bumper sticker reads: I + **N.Y.** (clubs)

Rapid Cooling of Andy's

Within an hour, Couri Hay from Team B knocks on my hotel-room door and murmurs the password. We drive in Couri's limo to the hospital. Our people—nurses, ward physician, attendants, security guards—are in total control of the ward. I wait down the hall with the perfusion team. And the substitute corpse, whom we Andy fans remember from the hoax in Salt Lake City.

At 3:45 A.M. EST we were notified that Andy was experiencing final, agonal respirations. At 3:59 AM, our man, Dr. Mellon Hitchcock, pronounced Andy legally dead.

The switching of corpses was performed swiftly. We immediately started cardiopulmonary support using a heart-lung resuscitator. We employed an esophageal gastric tube airway to secure Andy's airway against stomach secretions and ventilate him. Andy quickly regained colour and showed good chest expansion. He looked better, in fact, than he had since

1968, the year he was shot by Kynaston McShine, one of the hangers-on at his studio at MOMA.

Andy was then packed in ice and wheeled to the back elevator. We arrived at our mortuary on West 91st Street at approximately 4:30 A.M. and began administration of transport medications at 4:40 A.M. By 5:25 A.M. Andy was positioned on the mobile advanced life-support system, and surgery was underway to raise his femoral artery. In addition to his continuing good skin color, Andy's arterial blood was bright tomato red—indicating good oxygenation, and he had bright red capillary bleeding into the wound during surgery—all good signs. The coy blandness, pervasive and teasing in its appeal to the media, was gone! The deathless, albino pallor was gone!

I know, I think, how Andy felt at this moment.

Andy often experienced the stigmata of the insane science-fiction artist: alienation, blurred reality, despair. And here he lies, on the hibernation table, no longer looking like the last dandy. Flushing with cool blood, he is no longer the figure of the Artist as Nobody, but the Romantic Stereotype of the Artist—pinkish, involved, grappling with fate and transcendence.

He had already cooled to 29.3°C by the time bypass was started, and he rapidly cooled to a rectal temperature of 9°C over the next forty-five minutes. Imagine that!

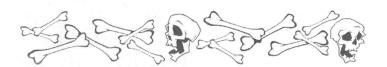

17

Celebrating Andy

A ndrew Warhola—Andy Warhol—was an American artist and a central figure in the movement known as pop art. After a successful career as a commercial illustrator, Warhol became famous worldwide for his work as a painter, avant-garde filmmaker, record producer, author, and public figure known for his membership in wildly diverse social circles that included bohemian street people, distinguished intellectuals, Hollywood celebrities and wealthy aristocrats.

Warhol has been the subject of numerous retrospective exhibitions, books, and feature and documentary films since his death in 1987.

Warhol coined the phrase "15 minutes of fame", which refers to the fleeting condition of celebrity that attaches to an object of media attention, then passes to some new object as soon as the public's attention span is exhausted.

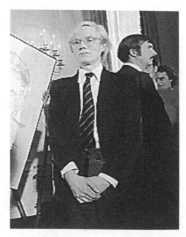

Dying is the most embarrassing thing that can ever happen to you, because someone's got to take care of all your details.

I never understood why when you died,
you didn't just vanish, everything could
just keep going on the way it was only
you just wouldn't be there. I always
thought I'd like my own tombstone to
be blank. No epitaph, and no name.
Well, actually, I'd like it to say 'figment.'

—ANDY WARHOL

Awaiting the Kiss
of Re-Animation

After supervising this delicate business, I am, un-
derstandably, thoroughly descoobied. So I went out
to an Eighth Avenue bar, which was noisy with kinky
sexual innuendoes. My whole head revolved around
laughter and crying, as my life turns down.

By the time I returned, blood washout and cryo-
protective perfusion had progressed nicely. At 8:43
A.M. I approved the decision to discontinue perfusion. Was this fair to Warhol? No, if you are among
those who think he had about five remarkable years
(1962-67) followed by a long down-slope decline into
money-making banality with his silk-screen editions
of dogs, famous Jews of the 20th Century, and Mer-
cedes Benzos. Yes, if you think that Andy was the
most important American artist since Jackson Pol-
lack. In any case, following the closure of the scalp
and chest incisions, Andy was placed inside two heavy
plastic bags and submerged in a silcone oil—Silcool—
bath had been precooled to 17°C.

Warhol's life force, uneven as it was lay in an
emotional fiction that contradicted the cold, fixed,
iconic surface, lowered at a rate of approximately 1°C
per hour to 17°C by gradual addition of dry ice to the
artificial—fake?—calm. My sense of Jamais Vue could
hardly be blamed on the MOMA curator who selected
these icons. A high-capacity pump was used to circu-
late the oil through a spray-bar assembly positioned
over the patient. This technique completely eliminat-
ed the "hot spots" and "cold spots" that have plagued
other artist's careers.

At 19:42 EST, the dewar was completely filled
with nitrogen, and Andy Warhol had entered long-
time hibernation! With him was put to rest gloomy
imaged of foreboding and death, like the skulls that
plagued the last years of his first, brief life.

That night, at the Gramercy Park Hotel, how I
envied Andy's cool tranquility as the hot fevered hand
of sleep sucked me down into the grave-ity of that
dark ground.

Andy Warhol is not dead. He hyphenated, a regal Ice
Queen in cool serendipity. His new life cycle has begun!
No thanks to medical science —and given a little bit of
luck, Andy will return to paint and paradox again!

At the grave site, the priest said a brief prayer
and sprinkled holy water three times over the casket.
Before it was lowered, Paige Powell dropped a copy of
Interview magazine, an Interview t-shirt, and a bottle
of Estee Lauder perfume into the grave. His tombstone
was a marble stone with Warhol's name and dates of
birth and death.

Public Celebration of Andy's Destruction

ANDY WARHOL
A Memorial Mass
www.findadeath.com
Wednesday, April 1, 1987 — St. Patrick's Cathedral

Prelude   *March of the Priest — The Magic Flute* — Mozart
Piano — Christopher O'Riley

Louange a l'Immortalite de Jesu — Oliver Messiaen
Cello — Carter Brey
Piano — Christopher O'Riley

Scriptures The Book of Wisdom 3: 1 — 9
Brigid Berlin

Speakers   John Richardson • Yoko Ono • Nicholas Love

Communion
Amazing Grace
Soloist — Latasha Spencer
www.findadeath.com
Prelude   *Recessional* — Ravel
Piano — Christopher O'Riley • Barbara Weintraub

Celebrant Father Anthony Dalla Villa, St. Patrick's Cathedral

John Grady, Director of Music, St. Patrick's Cathedral

A LESSER-KNOWN ELEMENT IN THE PORTRAIT OF ANDY WARHOL

Five hundred homeless and hungry New Yorkers will assemble on Easter Day at the Church of the Heavenly Rest, on Fifth Avenue at 90th Street. They will be served a delicious meal, and they will be treated as honored guests by some eighty volunteers. They will also be saddened by the absence of one who, with dedicated regularity, greeted them on Thanksgiving, Christmas and Easter. Andy poured coffee, served food and helped clean up. More than that he was a true friend to these friendless. He loved these nameless New Yorkers and they loved him back. We will pause to remember Andy this Easter, confident that he will be feasting with us at a Heavenly Banquet, because he had heard another Homeless Person who said: "I was hungry and you gave me food ... Truly, I say to you, as you did it to one of the least of these, any brothers and sisters, you did it to me."
The Reverend C. Hugh Hildesley, *Church of the Heavenly Rest*

Raphael I -$6.99 Andy Warhol 1985   Flowers to be donated to Mother Teresa -- Missionaries of Charity, The Department of Parks -- Forestry, and children's wards at various hospitals.

To everything there is a season,
A time to every purpose under heaven;
A time to be born, a time to die.

—ECCLESIASTES 3:1-2

Fifth Avenue in front of Saint Patrick's Cathedral was teeming with spectators and photographers and these last survivors of the human race who live in giant time-warp bubbles that they leave only to go to funerals, cremations, autopsies, and airplane crashes. They were lined up behind police fences, gaping at celebrities talking and grinning at the wide-eyed cameras celebrating the destruction of Andy's precious tissues—Or so they hoped!

The large doors of Saint Patrick's Cathedral opened this time portal into the Muddle Ages, high Gothic arches designed to dwarf the spirit of us individual quarks. Inside, this organist is playing, not Lower Eastside punk rock, not Velvet Underground, but Bach!

People file in with unhappy expressions. Young men with rainbow-dyed hair looking uncomfortable in suits and ties. And all this for a barbaric tissue-destruction ceremony. I can no longer remain silent when the people I love wind up in squirm holes and cremation barbecues.

Homage to the Maggots.
The Dread Sign of Crucifixion.
The Clown of Thorns

Orthodox Catholic witchcraft rituals begin predictably. The dread Sign of the Cross! The ominous kneeling in submission. Meanwhile, the clerical aliens quietly observing the humans, unsmiling in black-cloth (!) garments, family and friends sitting in peaceful twisted apathetic conformity. Don't be fooled

by them, these Catholic-Jewish-Islamaniacs who sit
brooding silently in darkened stone buildings. Behind
their frozen faces they are thinking about their loved
ones in the grave.

Don't be fooled by this fake Bible-Talmud-Koran
piety. Their Holy Books are male-order catalogues of
death worship. Their minds are busy thinking about
the maggots eating the flesh and brains (souls) of
their presumed loved ones. Or about the cruel oven
flames—dials turned to roast!—crackling the skins of
their dearly departed. Do you seriously think that they
can repress, just ignore the culinary facts? Not hear
the squishing noises of the maggots breeding cheerily
in the tissues of their sincerely departeds? The more
honest of these mourners are probably pondering
their own fate that awaits them in the fire and worms
departments.

The grisly papist plot crumbles to Gothic horror!
To put it charitably, Andy's funeral in Saint Patrick's
Cathedral is not an immortalist commercial. This
weird ritual demonstrates that We cannot escape
Their mortal coil. The semiotic message is clear.
Everything in this in mediaeval stone castle warns
us it is folly for individuals to seek immortality except through faith in one of the three Mediterranean
monotheistic mafias.

Would Andy Let Alien Priests Send Him Packing, Soul and Bones, to the Maggot Farm?

Our little, silver-haired pal, solemn, socially in-
secure, East European waif from Pittsburgh got the
point. Andy understood the cold, mechanical imper-
sonality of the industrial culture. Didn't he just blow
into the Big Applesauce factory from Pittsburgh, PA,
and call himself the Pope of Pop? Call his studio the
Factory? Send a reasonable facsimile, silver-wigged
model of himself around to give Warhol lectures at
colleges? Enter the Campbell Soup contest? Paint
reasonable facsimiles of soup-can labels and Marilyn
Monroes to win gigantic cash prizes? And admission
to correspondence art schools?

Death is it—the moment we've all been
waiting for—the last and singularly most
important even we will all have on our
resumes. How you die will speak vol-
umes about how you lived.

—TIMOTHY LEARY
Design for Dying

You think this crafty fox would let them pack him,
brain and bones, in a factory carton for easy delivery
to the maggot farm? Can you possibly think that Andy
Warhol would allow this public snuffing of his essence
by black-garbed minions of the cardinal? Who, come
to think of it, never tended to hang out at the Factory
and the office of *Interview* magazine.

Andy Invites You to His Re-Birthday Party

I understand that members of the Alcor Cryonics Foundation and thoughtful people around the four worlds who know about the hibernation of Walt Disney and Andy Warhol are celebrating and drinking toasts to the brave team who snatched Andy, literally, from the mouths of the maggots.

I also understand that some members of the Alcor Foundation, being of the very sincere, sober, scientific extraction, are concerned that a person of my colorful reputation could undermine Alcor's respectability and credibility. Particularly since disrespectability and incredibility are my predestined career goals in life.

I worry, myself, that since Alcor's important work is the ultimate threat to religious and political control, the last thing needed is to take on the negative baggage of a notorious jet set victim of the *National Enquirer* mentality.

Then I remember that to be a member of Alcor is to elect oneself as part of a noble band of heroes who are about to save humanity from the horror of involuntary, irreversible, metabolic coma. And therefore Alcor members are tolerant of my eccentricity, knowing it is a hard job, in this weirdo, death-worshipping culture, to be continually recast in these "Oscar Wilde" sequels.

By the way! Andy asked me to especially invite all of you to his re-animation party. Andy was very insistent that, at the glorious moment of re-animation, when his friends gather around his hibernation crystal, that you be there. Either in the ice tray or on the hoof. Write the Alcor Foundation if you have any questions about transportation to the party. "PLAN A HEAD" is our motto!

The gray-haired black man warned Andy, as he did me and Bill Burroughs: Stay our of prisons and hospitals, son. Avoid ministers, priests, and rabbis. All they got is the key to the shit house. And promise me, boy, you will never wear the badge of a lawman. And if you do end up serving time in the white man's body factories—complete service from womb to tomb, join a gang of friends that will cover for you. And if you have to be admitted to the disposal room—planned obsolescence is their marketing strategy, just be sure you've got friends hanging around, watching over you day and night, lest someone make off with your beloved albino animal skin. And contents thereof.

It seems very likely that your final trip will last a subjective eternity, and that how you navigate that final trip will determine whether you have an ecstatic or a hellish experience. It also seems very likely that the final trip is very similar to psychedelic drug experiences.

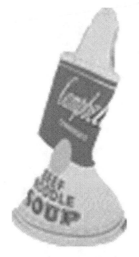

—TIMOTHY LEARY
Design for Dying

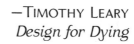

18

Timothy Leary's 23 Skidoo

Contributed by

Michael David Segel

Shortly after Timothy's death, his ashes were divided up between a few friends and family members. Because my sister then lived back East, I picked some up for her as well. While deciding whether or not to mail the ashes to her, the following paranoid scenario took over . . .

The Associated Press

LOS ANGELES – The first of many arrests was make Thursday, following a raid carried out by a task force comprised of several federal agencies and spearheaded by the Federal Bureau of Investigation. Taken into custody were two members of what is believed to be a nationwide, family-run cartel.

The raid followed the discovery by a United States Postal Inspector of a package containing approximately two ounces of a course, grayish powder. The powder, the suspects insist, is the cremated remains of World-renown philosopher Dr. Timothy Leary. The ashes, however, have since tested positive for a number of controlled substances, acquired evidently over Dr. Leary's lifetime.

The suspects are being held without bail, pending arraignment, on multiple felony counts including possession, possession with intent to distribute and transportation of controlled substances across state lines. Dr. Leary's ashes were seized by Federal Agents from both the Drug Enforcement Agency and the Bureau of Alcohol, Tobacco and Firearms. Neither agency would divulge their estimated street value.

Special Agent J. Orange of the FBI was quoted as saying, "We won't stop here. We will determine who else has these psycho-active remains in their possession. We will hut them down and we will seize their contraband." He continues, "We fully intend to kick their ashes."

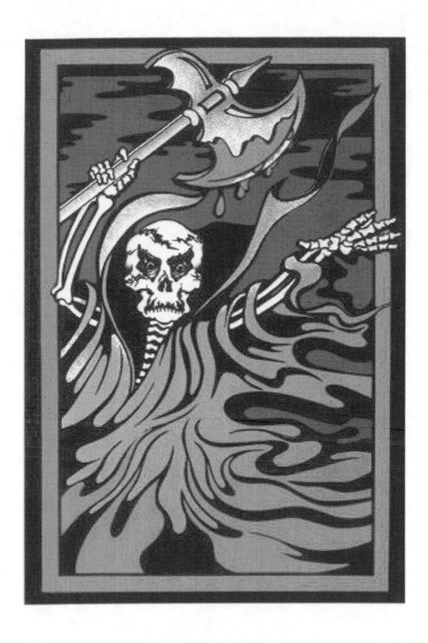

Timothy Leary (1920-1996) was a
world-renowned psychologist, a defrocked
Harvard professor, a relentless champion
of individual freedom, a stand-up philosopher, a Federal "criminal," and a leading
light of counterculture thinking.

Question Authority
Think for Yourself
Reboot Your Brain

Ronin Books for Independent

THE FIGUTIVE PHILOSOPHER..Leary/FIGPHI $12.95 __
From Harvard Professor to fugitive—the amazing story.

PSYCHEDELIC PRAYERS..Leary/PSYPRA $12.95 __
Guide to transcendental experience based on Tao Te Ching

PSYCHEDELIC PRAYERS—Keepsake Edition........Leary/PSYPRA-C $20.00 __
Hard cover—makes a great gift for 60s enthusiast

HIGH PRIEST...Leary/HIGPRI $19.95 __
Acid trips lead by Huxley, Ginsburg, Burroughs, Ram Dass and other 60s gurus

HIGH PRIEST—Collector's Edition............................Leary/HIGPRI-C $100.00 __
Limited edition in hard cover, numbered and signed by Timothy Leary

POLITICS OF ECSTASY...Leary/POLECS $14.95 __
Classic, the book that got Leary called the "most dangerous man in America"

CHANGE YOUR BRAIN..........................:..........................Leary/CHAYOU $12.95 __
Brain change is more taboo than sex and why

DISCORDIA...DISCORD $14.00 __
Parody of religion based upon Eris, goddess of chaos & confusion.

EVOULTIONARY AGENTS:...Leary/EVOAGE $12.95 __
Leary's future history. Why the only smart thing to do is to get smarter.

POLITICS OF SELF-DETERMINATION.........................Leary/POLSEL $12.95 __
Leary's pre-Harvard years & his *real* claim to fame that got him to Harvard.

MUSINGS ON HUMAN METAMORPHOSES ....Leary/MUSING $12.95 __
Spin psychology. Mutants and malcontents migrate first. The only place to go is up!

CYBERPUNKS CYBERFREEDOM.............................Leary/CUBPUN $12.95 __
Reboot your brain. Change reality screens.

POLITICS OF PSYCHOPHARMOCOLOGY.................Leary/POLPSY $12.95 __
Story of Tim's persecution for his ideas including interrogation by Teddy Kennedy.

CHAOS AND CYBER CULTURE..................................Leary/CHACYB $29.95 __
Cyberpunk manifesto on designing chaos and fashioning personal disorders

START YOUR OWN RELIGION..................................... Leary/STAREL $14.00 __
Gather your cult, write your own New Testament, select your sacrament.

Books prices: SUBTOTAL $_____

CA customers add sales tax 8.75% _____

BASIC SHIPPING: (All orders)   **$6.00**

PLUS SHIPPING: USA+$1/bk, Canada+$2/bk, Europe+$6/bk, Pacific+$8/bk _____

Books + Tax + Basic shipping + Shipping per book: TOTAL $_____

Check/MO payable to **Ronin Publishing**

MC __ Visa __ Discover __ Exp date _ _ / _ _ card #:___/___/___/___

Signature _____

Ronin Publishing, Inc • Box 22900 • Oakland, CA 94609
Ph:800/858.2665 • Fax:510/420-3672
www.roninpub.com for online catalog
Price & availability subject to change without notice

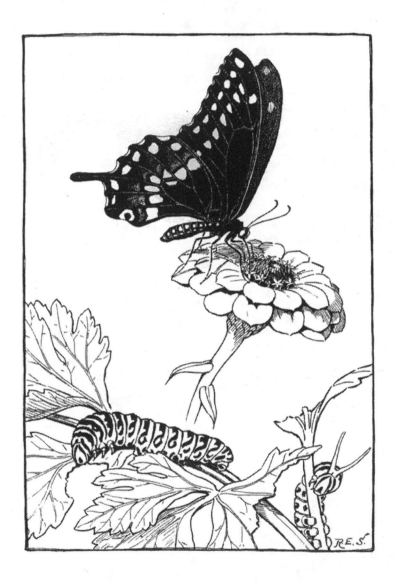